Postgraduate Orthopaedics: MCQs and EMQs for the FRCS (Tr & Orth)

D1430102

Postgraduate Orthopaedics: MCQs and EMQs for the FRCS (Tr & Orth)

Edited by

Kesavan Sri-Ram, BSc, MRCS (Eng), FRCS (Tr & Orth)
Senior Arthroplasty Fellow, Royal National Orthopaedic Hospital and Wycombe Hospital, UK

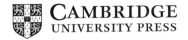

CAMBRIDGE
UNIVERSITY PRESS

CAMBRIDGE UNIVERSITY PRESS
Cambridge, New York, Melbourne, Madrid, Cape Town,
Singapore, São Paulo, Delhi, Tokyo, Mexico City

Cambridge University Press
The Edinburgh Building, Cambridge CB2 8RU, UK

Published in the United States of America by
Cambridge University Press, New York

www.cambridge.org
Information on this title: www.cambridge.org/9780521184717

First published 2012

Printed in the United Kingdom at the University Press, Cambridge

A catalogue record for this publication is available from the British Library

Library of Congress Cataloging-in-Publication Data

Postgraduate orthopaedics : MCQS and EMQS for the FRCS (Tr & Orth) /
edited by Kesavan Sri-Ram.
   p.   ;   cm.
Includes bibliographical references and index.
ISBN 978-0-521-18471-7 (Paperback)
I. Sri-Ram, Kesavan.
[DNLM: 1.   Orthopedic Procedures–Examination Questions.   WE 18.2]
LC classification not assigned
617′.9076–dc23
                                                                                    2011029387

ISBN 978-0-521-18471-7 Paperback

For Sharmili

Contents

Contributors

Mr Rajiv A. Bajekal, MS (Orth), ChM (Orth), FRCS (Orth)
Consultant Orthopaedic Surgeon, Barnet Hospital, London

Professor Tim W.R. Briggs, MD (Res), MCh (Orth), FRCS
Professor of Orthopaedic Surgery and Orthopaedic Oncology, Royal National Orthopaedic Hospital, Stanmore

Mr Zaher Dannawi, FRCS (Tr & Orth)
Spinal Fellow, Royal National Orthopaedic Hospital, Stanmore

Miss Deborah M. Eastwood FRCS
Consultant Orthopaedic Surgeon, Royal National Orthopaedic Hospital, Stanmore

Mr Dennis Edwards, FRCS (Orth)
Consultant Orthopaedic Surgeon, Cambridge University NHS Trust, Cambridge

Mr Russell Hawkins, FRCS (Tr & Orth)
Specialist Registrar in Trauma and Orthopaedic Surgery, Royal National Orthopaedic Hospital, Stanmore

Miss Deborah S. Higgs, MBBS, FRCS (Tr & Orth)
Consultant Shoulder and Elbow Surgeon, Royal National Orthopaedic Hospital, Stanmore

Mr Maxim Horwitz, FRCS (Tr & Orth)
Locum Consultant Orthopaedic and Hand Surgeon, St Mary's Hospital, Imperial College Healthcare NHS Trust, London

Mr Phil Kerr, FRCS
Consultant Orthopaedic Surgeon, Lister Hospital, Stevenage

Mr Simon Lambert, BSc, FRCS, FRCS Ed (Orth)
Consultant Shoulder and Elbow Surgeon, Royal National Orthopaedic Hospital, Stanmore

Mr Danyal H. Nawabi, BM, MA, MRCS (Eng), FRCS (Tr & Orth)
Specialist Registrar in Trauma and Orthopaedic Surgery, Royal National Orthopaedic Hospital, Stanmore

Mr Andrew 'Fred' Robinson, BSc, FRCS (Orth)
Consultant Foot and Ankle Surgeon, Cambridge University NHS Trust, Cambridge

Mr Ben Rudge, FRCS (Tr & Orth)
Specialist Registrar in Trauma and Orthopaedic Surgery, Whittington Hospital, London

Mr Nashat Ahmad Siddiqui, FRCS (Tr & Orth)
Specialist Registrar in Trauma and Orthopaedic Surgery, Royal Free Hospital, London

Mr John A. Skinner, FRCS (Orth)
Consultant Orthopaedic Surgeon, Royal National Orthopaedic Hospital, Stanmore

Mr Elliot Sorene, MBBS, FRCS (Tr & Orth), EDHS
Consultant Orthopaedic and Hand Surgeon, University College London Hospital, London

Mr Kesavan Sri-Ram, BSc, MRCS (Eng), FRCS (Tr & Orth)
Senior Arthroplasty Fellow, Wycombe Hospital, Wycombe and Royal National Orthopaedic Hospital, Stanmore

Mr Howard Ware, FRCS (Orth)
Consultant Orthopaedic Surgeon, Wellington Knee Surgery Unit, London and Chase Farm Hospital, Enfield

Mr Paul Whittingham-Jones, FRCS (Tr & Orth)
Specialist Registrar in Trauma and Orthopaedic Surgery, Royal National Orthopaedic Hospital, Stanmore

Foreword

The biggest hurdle for the modern orthopaedic trainee is passing the FRCS (Tr & Orth) exit examination. Practice is necessary when preparing for any examination, and the written component of the FRCS (Tr & Orth) is no exception. However, this does need to be focused.

So why another book? These MCQs and EMQs are divided according to subspecialty so the questions can easily be used as part of a revision plan.

Detailed explanations are given in the answers making this a revision guide by topic as well as practice with the question-and-answer format.

Written by surgeons with recent examination experience, this book features both styles of exam questions and covers the topics in the FRCS (Tr & Orth) syllabus.

Mr Barry Ferris MS FRCS
Consultant Orthopaedic Surgeon
Barnet Hospital, London

Preface

Examinations are always a nuisance, especially as you enter more mature years. Studying becomes less natural and more tedious. Thankfully, the FRCS (Tr & Orth) examination is just about orthopaedics, and so some of the knowledge required would hopefully be second nature. However, MCQ and EMQ examinations always tend to ask about less obvious topics, which do not always feature in routine practice, and this is no different with the FRCS (Tr & Orth).

When many of the authors were preparing for their examination, there was a distinct shortage of practice questions. The vast majority related to American examinations, and our experience was that these are very different to the questions in the British examination.

The aim of this book, therefore, is to provide the candidate with a feel of the standard of questions in the examination. Divided into subspecialty chapters, the book contains both MCQs and EMQs in the same format as the FRCS (Tr & Orth), with many of the topics encountered in the actual examination by the authors. Each chapter is complete with explanations to provide the required knowledge and selected references for further reading.

Although a great deal of work is required to pass this examination, it is hoped that this book provides not only knowledge, but also some reassurance that the process will go smoothly.

Kesavan Sri-Ram

Acknowledgements

I'm very grateful for all the authors who have found time in busy schedules to write the chapters and keep to the deadlines (ish!). Many of the authors were part of my 'study group', and were instrumental in me getting through the FRCS. I am also grateful for the training experiences with every consultant I have had the privilege to work for and be trained by; these, without exception, have been excellent.

I would like to thank Nick and Joanna at Cambridge University Press for all their help during the entire process of composing this book, right from the initial proposal through to the final editing.

My appreciation for the support from friends and family, especially my parents, goes without saying, but my biggest thank you is to my wife, Sharmili, and girls, Alisha, Riya and Shrina, who allowed me enough time in my 'office' to put this book together.

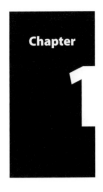

Chapter

1

Introduction

Kesavan Sri-Ram

The exam format

The written component of the FRCS (Tr & Orth) examination (referred to as Section 1) comprises of multiple choice questions (MCQs; also known as single best answer) and extended matching questions (EMQs; also known as extended matching items). There are usually three sittings of this examination each year.

There are two papers held on the same day:

Paper 1 –	110 MCQs
	2 hours 15 minutes
	First 12 questions relate to a paper
	First 15 minutes is for reading the paper only (questions cannot be read)
Paper 2 –	135 EMQs (i.e. 3 × 45)
	2 hours 30 minutes*

* The time limit was initially 2 hours, but was increased after a few sittings.

Traditionally, candidates filled out standard computer-read MCQ answer sheets, but more recently, the intercollegiate specialty board (ISB) has introduced computer-based testing for the written examination. Full details are available on the ISB website (http://www.intercollegiate.org.uk) and are provided to all candidates.

The MCQs

The first 12 questions are based on an orthopaedic article. From experience, it seems that this is usually a short article, with straightforward methodology and statistics. The questions relating to the article are concerned with the study design, methods, results and statistics, but also the core knowledge relating to the article's subject. The first question is usually related to the type of study (e.g. randomized controlled trail, prospective cohort study, case–control study, retrospective cohort study or case series) so it is worth learning these well to guarantee one mark.

A few examples of articles used in previous examinations are:

Ohly NE, Murray IR, Keating JF. Revision anterior cruciate ligament reconstruction: timing of surgery and the incidence of meniscal tears and degenerative change. *J Bone Joint Surg Br* 2007; **89**(8): 1051–4.

Postgraduate Orthopaedics, ed. Kesavan Sri-Ram. Published by Cambridge University Press.
© Cambridge University Press 2012.

Shetty AA, Tindall AJ, James KD, Relwani J, Fernando KW. Accuracy of hand-held ultrasound scanning in detecting meniscal tears. *J Bone Joint Surg Br* 2008; **90**(8): 1045–8.

Tang WC, Henderson IJ. High tibial osteotomy: long term survival analysis and patients' perspective. *Knee* 2005; **12**(6): 410–13.

Wraighte PJ, Howard PW. Femoral impaction bone allografting with an Exeter cemented collarless, polished, tapered stem in revision hip replacement: a mean follow-up of 10.5 years. *J Bone Joint Surg Br* 2008; **90**(8): 1000–4.

The remaining MCQs test core knowledge. There are many questions relating to anatomy and exposures. There are many clinical questions and generally, controversial topics are avoided. It should be noted that the style of questions are very different to those used for United States examinations (although many of the topics are common) and this should be borne in mind when using such questions for practice.

The EMQs

Each set of three EMQs will refer to a particular topic, and there may be up to 15 options. Each question will have the instruction similar to:

'Which of the options above is best described in each of the following statements? Each option may be used once, more than once or not at all.'

The questions are often clinical scenarios and there are usually one or two key words which will direct you to the answer.

General advice

Unfortunately, the examination is a stressful experience. However, the following advice may be helpful during the process:

- Both papers are long, and time really is constrained; therefore go fast.
- The first 12 questions in the MCQ paper can take a long time as you need to refer back to the article; it is worth setting a time limit for these and moving on if delayed.
- There is no negative marking, and so an answer must be offered for each question.
- If an answer is not known, do not leave a gap, in case there is no time to come back to that question.
- Read the MCQs carefully; in particular watch out for requests for the incorrect statement (i.e. which of the following is incorrect regarding . . .)
- Do not read through all of the options for the EMQs; instead, read the question and find the answer (i.e. you should ideally know the answer before seeing it in the options provided).

Preparation

Like many things in life, preparation is the key to success. Although most of the knowledge would have been acquired during training, the syllabus is very extensive, and so, for the examination, needs to be learned, and needs plenty of time.

Unlike the old examination, which took place over a few days, the new format has the written component often a few months before the clinical and vivas. As a result, one can focus one's revision accordingly. It is probably best to start revising at least six months before the examination, and have a revision plan.

There are several good texts which help the process. Many candidates rely, rightly, on Miller's *Review of Orthopaedics*. In addition, one should possess good texts for basic science, anatomy and surgical exposures.

Practising MCQs is very important, not only to reinforce the knowledge, but also to get a feel for the time restriction. More recently, UKITE (UK in Training Exams) is being used by trainees and adopted by some regions as part of annual assessment. This process would provide very good preparation for the written paper.

Finally, as with the clinical component of the examination, a study group is incredibly helpful for the written paper and this was certainly the case for many of the authors!

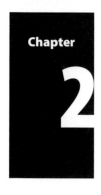

Chapter 2

Hand and wrist: Questions

Maxim Horwitz and Elliot Sorene

MCQs

1. **Which of the following is not a cause of a swan neck deformity?**
   a. Mallet deformity.
   b. Flexor tendon tenosynovitis.
   c. Volar plate rupture.
   d. Central slip rupture.
   e. Lateral band subluxation.

2. **When performing a replant of an amputated finger, which of the following is the correct order of surgery?**
   a. Bone, Artery, Extensor, Flexor, Nerve, Vein.
   b. Artery, Bone, Vein, Extensor, Flexor, Nerve.
   c. Artery, Bone, Extensor, Flexor, Vein, Nerve.
   d. Bone, Extensor, Flexor, Artery, Nerve, Vein.
   e. Bone, Extensor, Flexor, Artery, Vein, Nerve.

3. **When performing flexor tendon repair, which of the following pulleys must be preserved?**
   a. A2 and A4.
   b. A2 only.
   c. A2 and C2.
   d. A2 and A3.
   e. A3 only.

4. **A Stener lesion is significant because?**
   a. Adductor aponeurosis interposition between the proximally based avulsed ligament impairs ligament healing.
   b. Adductor aponeurosis interposition between the distally based avulsed ligament impairs ligament healing.
   c. Skiing is an increasingly popular sport.
   d. It involves partial and complete ulnar collateral ligament rupture.
   e. It is associated with a fleck sign on the X-ray.

Postgraduate Orthopaedics, ed. Kesavan Sri-Ram. Published by Cambridge University Press.
© Cambridge University Press 2012.

5. **Which of the following regarding metacarpal neck fractures is true?**
   a. Up to 35° of angulation of the index and middle finger can be accepted.
   b. Up to 40° of angulation of the little and ring finger can be accepted.
   c. Metacarpal neck fractures should never be operated upon unless it is an open injury.
   d. The Jahss position is the correct position to immobilize a manipulated metacarpal neck fracture.
   e. Up to 15° of angulation of the index and middle finger can be accepted.

6. **When reducing a Smith's or volar Barton's fracture, the reduction manoeuvre should include?**
   a. Supination only.
   b. Extension only.
   c. Extension and supination.
   d. Extension and pronation.
   e. Flexion and supination.

7. **A 22-year-old medical student was slightly intoxicated and fell onto his extended wrist while his forearm was pronated. He has pain and a clicking sensation on the ulnar side of his wrist. X-rays and nerve conduction studies are normal. The most likely diagnosis is?**
   a. Scapholunate dissociation.
   b. Hook of hamate fracture.
   c. Triangular fibrocartilage complex (TFCC) tear.
   d. Piso-triquetral subluxation.
   e. Extensor carpi ulnaris (ECU) subluxation.

8. **If a 28-year-old male motorbiker had a complex distal radius fracture (volar fixation required) and acute severe carpal tunnel syndrome, which of the following surgical approaches would be correct?**
   a. Perform a Henry's approach and a separate, very ulnar carpal tunnel incision.
   b. Observe the carpal tunnel syndrome for 48 hours after surgery.
   c. Perform a Henry's approach and a separate carpal tunnel incision.
   d. Continue Henry's approach across the wrist with an S curve and decompress the carpal tunnel.
   e. Continue Henry's approach across the wrist and decompress the carpal tunnel.

9. **Which of the following is not a sign of an unstable scaphoid fracture?**
   a. Vertical oblique fracture.
   b. Comminuted fracture.
   c. >1 mm displacement.
   d. Associated perilunate injury.
   e. Scapholunate angle <60°.

10. **In Wartenburg syndrome the compression takes place between?**
    a. Brachioradialis and extensor carpi radialis longus (ECRL) in pronation.
    b. Brachioradialis and ECRL in supination.
    c. ECRL and extensor carpi radialis brevis (ECRB).

    d. Abductor pollicis longus (APL), extensor pollicis brevis (EPB) and ECRL, ECRB.

    e. Brachioradialis and flexor carpi radialis (FCR).

11. **A patient presents with pain and cold insensitivity at the fingertip. There is a bluish discolouration under the nail. The most likely diagnosis is?**

    a. Neurofibroma.

    b. Glomus tumour.

    c. Turret tumour.

    d. Epithelioid sarcoma.

    e. Raynaud's disease.

12. **The following are all good prognosis after nerve injury except?**

    a. Young age.

    b. Low velocity injury.

    c. Sharp (knife) injury.

    d. Proximal injury.

    e. Early exploration.

13. **All of the following make up the spiral cord except?**

    a. Grayson's ligaments.

    b. Spiral band.

    c. Lateral sheet.

    d. Natatory ligament.

    e. Pretendinous band.

14. **Which of the following is not a poor prognostic indicator in traumatic brachial plexus injury?**

    a. Horner's sign.

    b. Transverse process fracture.

    c. Empty sheaths on MRI scan.

    d. Diaphragmatic flattening on inspiration/expiration X-rays.

    e. No sensation from tip of acromion to tip of fingers.

15. **Which of the following is a rule of tendon transfer?**

    a. The donor muscle must be at least MRC grade 3.

    b. Joints can have 50% maximum contracture.

    c. Tendon pull must be synergistic.

    d. Line of pull should be orthogonal.

    e. Tendon excursions of the finger extensors is longer than the flexors.

16. **A 56-year-old obese man presents with a painless deterioration in bilateral hand function. Initially it was the metacarpophalangeal (MCP) and proximal interphalangeal (PIP) joints that were involved and now it is the distal interphalangeal (DIP) joints. He has thick tight skin and a positive prayer sign. The most likely disease is?**

    a. Gout.

    b. Osteoarthritis.

    c. Rheumatoid arthritis.

d. Scleroderma.

e. Diabetic cheirarthropathy.

17. A 38-year-old man presents with dorsal wrist pain. He has a stiff wrist with very limited range of motion and can't work as a mechanic. Plain films reveal Grade IV Kienbock's disease. He should be treated with?

a. Proximal row carpectomy.

b. Wrist replacement.

c. Curettage and vascularized pronator quadratus graft.

d. Radial shortening.

e. Wrist arthrodesis.

18. A 41-year-old woman sustained a distal radius fracture whilst hiking in the Andes. It was treated in plaster by a local missionary doctor and went on to malunion. She presents with ulnar-sided pain and on examination she impacts on the ulnar side, with a negative grind test at the distal radioulnar joint (DRUJ). The best treatment would be?

a. Ulnar shortening osteotomy.

b. Darrach procedure.

c. Sauve–Kapandji procedure.

d. Arthroscopic debridement of DRUJ.

e. Distal ulnar head implant arthroplasty.

19. Which of the following is not true of Dupuytren's disease?

a. The long-term recurrence rate is 50%.

b. Painful nodules are an indication for surgery.

c. Metacarpophalangeal joint (MCPJ) contracture of greater than 30° is an indication for surgery.

d. Myofibroblasts are the offending cells in the aetiology of the disease.

e. Concomitant carpal tunnel release increases incidence of post-operative flare.

20. A 17-year-old snowboarder fell onto his outstretched pronated hand. He presents with ongoing ulnar-sided wrist pain. He is tender over the ulnar fovea and has no click. The distal radioulnar joint (DRUJ) is stable. Plain films are normal and a MR arthrogram show a triangular fibrocartilage complex (TFCC) defect adjacent to the ulna. How is this classified according to the Palmer classification?

a. Class 2A lesion.

b. Class 1A lesion.

c. Class 2B lesion.

d. Class 1B lesion.

e. Class 1C lesion.

21. A 16-year-old girl had multiple fractures in her forearm and hand. One year later after fracture healing she presents with trouble gripping things. When the metacarpophalangeal (MCP) joint is extended you cannot passively flex the proximal interphalangeal (PIP) joint. When the MCP joint is flexed it is possible to passively flex the PIP joint. Her extensors are at a good length. Which of the following is incorrect?

7

a. She has an intrinsic plus hand.
b. She has a claw hand.
c. She has a positive Bunnell test.
d. She has a likely positive Bouviere effect.
e. There is an imbalance between the intrinsic and extrinsic muscles.

22. A 23-year-old cricketer had an avulsion of the flexor digitorum profundus (FDP) tendon of his ring finger. This was diagnosed early and despite proximal migration he had it reinserted with a button technique. Six months later he complains that he can't close his fingers tightly over a cricket ball. This problem is?
a. Lumbrical plus effect.
b. Swan neck deformity.
c. Quadrigia effect.
d. Intrinsic tightness.
e. Chronic mallet finger.

23. Which of the following is true regarding a Mayfield Stage I injury?
a. There is not always a scaphoid fracture.
b. There is a lunotriquetral ligament injury.
c. The lunate is extruded.
d. There is a radio-scapho-capitate ligament detachment.
e. There is a perilunate dislocation.

24. A 23-year-old was intoxicated at a wedding and fell through a glass window. He presents to the emergency department with a radial wrist laceration with arterial bleeding. With regards to the timing of surgery the major blood supply to the hand is provided by which of the following?
a. Deep branch of the radial artery.
b. Radial artery.
c. Deep palmar arch.
d. Superficial palmar arch.
e. Interosseous artery.

25. A 41-year-old man presents with a swelling at the level of his distal interphalangeal (DIP) joint on his right middle finger. What is the most likely diagnosis?
a. Epidermoid cyst.
b. Keratoacanthoma.
c. Mucoid cyst.
d. Epithelioid tumour.
e. Sebaceous cyst.

26. Which of the following is not a recognized treatment for carpal tunnel syndrome?
a. Nerve stimulation therapy.
b. Steroid injection.
c. One-portal endoscopic surgical release.
d. Two-portal endoscopic surgical release.
e. Yoga.

27. **All of the following contribute to the wrist and hand deformity in rheumatoid arthritis except?**
    a. Volar subluxation of the extensor carpi ulnaris (ECU).
    b. Radio-scapho-capitate ligament failure.
    c. Scaphoid extension.
    d. Supination of the carpus on the forearm.
    e. Distal radioulnar joint (DRUJ) destruction.

28. **A 13-year-old boy is referred to you after a trivial fall onto his elbow. Radiographs reveal a dislocated radial head. He does not have much pain. His mother says she has always had joint pains with abnormal knee caps. She keeps pointing to her knees in an excited manner with long fake nails. The most likely diagnosis is?**
    a. Marfan syndrome.
    b. Monteggia Bado injury.
    c. Generalized ligamentous laxity.
    d. Ehlers–Danlos syndrome.
    e. Nail patella syndrome.

29. **A 43-year-old woman presents with decreased digital flexion and an injury in Zone 2 of her left hand. On exploration what percentage laceration of the flexor tendon would you repair?**
    a. 40%.
    b. 25%.
    c. 45%.
    d. 50%.
    e. 35%.

30. **With regards to radioulnar limb formation and the zone of polarizing activity, defects in which protein will result in duplication of digits?**
    a. Fibroblast growth factor.
    b. Sonic hedgehog protein.
    c. LMX1.
    d. Transforming growth factor.
    e. Cartilage-derived morphogenetic protein.

EMQs

1. **Causes of wrist pain**
   a. De Quervain's disease
   b. Chronic triangular fibrocartilage complex (TFCC) lesion with sigmoid notch detachment
   c. Extensor carpi ulnaris (ECU) subluxation and tenosynovitis
   d. Intersection syndrome
   e. Late tendon rupture after distal radius fracture
   f. Vaughn-Jackson syndrome
   g. Extensor digitorum communis (EDC) to ring finger subluxation
   h. Wartenburg syndrome

Which of the options above is best described in each of the following statements? Each option may be used once, more than once or not at all.
   1. A male 27-year-old university rower who plays the drums complains of wrist pain.
   2. A 43-year-old woman on anti-tumour necrosis factor (anti-TNF) medication reports that her hand function has deteriorated dramatically.
   3. A 23-year-old woman presents with radial-sided wrist pain. Her full-time job is caring for her 6-month-old baby and 2-year-old toddler.

2. **Infections in the hand**
   a. Orf virus
   b. *Staphylococcus aureus*
   c. Clostridia and Group A β-streptococci
   d. Herpes simplex virus type 1
   e. *Candida albicans*
   f. *Mycobacterium marinum*
   g. *Eikenella corrodens*
   h. *Pasteurella multocida*

Which of the options above is best described in each of the following statements? Each option may be used once, more than once or not at all.
   1. A 26-year-old presents to the emergency department with a small laceration over his index metacarpal of his right hand. It is swollen with pus draining. History relates to a punching incident.
   2. A dentist presents with recurrent vesicles on the fingers and pain.
   3. A 65-year-old woman was bitten by a cat on the dorsum of the left wrist and now can't move the hand and has severe swelling and pain.

3. **Wound management**
   a. Cross finger flap
   b. Heterodigital island flap
   c. Terminalization
   d. Haematoma evacuation
   e. Nail bed repair and splint
   f. V-Y plasty (advancement)

g. Distal replant
h. Full thickness skin grafting

Which of the options above is best described in each of the following statements? Each option may be used once, more than once or not at all.
1. A 26-year-old chef cuts the tip of his finger with a sharp knife. There is no bone exposed, the wound is volar favourable and >1 cm is exposed.
2. A 42-year-old housewife minced the pulp of her index finger and there is a volar unfavourable wound with exposed bone >1 cm.
3. A gardener put his hand under the blade of a lawnmower. There is very little bone in the distal phalanx with an exposed ragged flexor digitorum profundus (FDP) tendon and no nail visible.

4. **Tumours of the hand**
   a. Malignant nerve sheath tumour
   b. Synovial
   c. Epithelioid
   d. Neurofibroma
   e. Schwannoma
   f. Ewing's
   g. Enchondroma
   h. Squamous cell carcinoma
   i. Pyogenic granuloma
   j. Sweat gland tumour

Which of the options above is best described in each of the following statements? Each option may be used once, more than once or not at all.
1. This is the most common soft tissue sarcoma of the hand.
2. This is the most common benign bone tumour and if multiple carries a 30% risk of sarcoma.
3. A lesion of the nerves that shells out like a pea from a pod.

5. **Inflammatory conditions**
   a. Rheumatoid arthritis
   b. Scleroderma
   c. Systemic lupus erythematosus
   d. Gout
   e. Amyloidosis
   f. Psoriasis
   g. Osteoarthritis
   h. Calcium pyrophosphate deposits

Which of the options above is best described in each of the following statements? Each option may be used once, more than once or not at all.
1. A 47-year-old with onycholysis and a 'pencil in cup' appearance of the fingers on X-ray presents with painful distal interphalangeal (DIP) joints.

2. A 52-year-old woman presents with subcutaneous calcinosis, Raynaud's phenomenon and painful fingers.
3. This 65-year-old man on renal dialysis presents with stiff painful fingers and one of the digits triggers. A research project has revealed β2 microglobulins in the soft tissues of his fingers.

6. Nerve compression
   a. Parsonage–Turner syndrome
   b. Posterior interosseous nerve palsy
   c. Pronator syndrome
   d. Radial tunnel syndrome
   e. Anterior interosseous nerve palsy
   f. Cubital tunnel syndrome
   g. Carpal tunnel syndrome
   h. Mannerfelt–Norman syndrome

Which of the options above is best described in each of the following statements? Each option may be used once, more than once or not at all.
   1. A 45-year-old man has a viral illness and then develops motor weakness in flexion of the thumb and index finger.
   2. A 25-year-old man has a weak pronator quadratus and a weak OK sign. An ultrasound reveals thick bicipital bursae.
   3. A 57-year-old woman with rheumatoid arthritis has a sudden inability to make the OK sign.

7. Surgical options
   a. Wrist fusion
   b. Lunotriquetral fusion
   c. Ulnar shortening
   d. Radial shortening
   e. Proximal row carpectomy
   f. Lunate excision
   g. Capitate lengthening

Which of the options above is best described in each of the following statements? Each option may be used once, more than once or not at all.
   1. A patient with dorsal wrist pain and an ulnar minus variance with Lichtman stage 3A disease.
   2. A patient with dorsal wrist pain and an ulnar minus variance with Lichtman stage 3B disease.
   3. A patient with dorsal wrist pain and an ulnar minus variance with Lichtman stage 4 disease.

8. Hand deformities
   a. Intrinsic plus hand
   b. Boutonnière deformity
   c. Pseudo-boutonnière deformity

    d. Swan neck deformity
    e. Intrinsic minus hand
    f. Quadrigia effect
    g. Lumbrical plus finger
    h. Caput ulnae wrist

Which of the options above is best described in each of the following statements? Each option may be used once, more than once or not at all.
    1. On metacarpophalangeal joint (MCPJ) extension there is less flexion of the proximal interphalangeal joint (PIPJ) than with passive flexion of the MCPJ.
    2. Tendons adjacent to an injured finger (usually flexor tendon) don't flex owing to a shared muscle belly.
    3. Central slip rupture leads to this condition.

9. Injuries around the wrist
    a. Dorsal wrist ganglion
    b. Hamate hook fracture
    c. Piso-triquetral arthritis
    d. Scapho-trapezio-trapezoid (STT) osteoarthritis
    e. Scaphoid non-union advanced collapse
    f. Distal radioulnar joint osteoarthritis
    g. Ulnocarpal abutment
    h. Extensor carpi ulnaris tendonitis
    i. De Quervain's disease
    j. First carpometacarpal osteoarthritis
    k. Scaphoid lunate advanced collapse
    l. Triangular fibrocartilage complex (TFCC) injury

Which of the options above is best described in each of the following statements? Each option may be used once, more than once or not at all.
    1. A 22-year-old medical student presents 3 weeks after falling onto his hand after a few drinks at a party. He says his little finger feels a bit numb.
    2. A 62-year-old woman presents 6 months after a Colles fracture that was treated in plaster. Radiographs reveal a loss of radial height (2+ ulnar positive).
    3. A 29-year-old with radial-sided wrist pain has a positive ring sign on X-ray with an increased scapholunate angle.

10. Surgery for the wrist
    a. Wrist fusion with AO fusion plate
    b. Radio-scapholunate fusion
    c. Scaphoidectomy and four-corner fusion
    d. Proximal row carpectomy
    e. Arthroscopic debridement
    f. Scapholunate ligament reconstruction
    g. Lunotriquetral arthrodesis
    h. Triquetral-hamate fusion

Which of the options above is best described in each of the following statements? Each option may be used once, more than once or not at all.

1. A 28-year-old female had a comminuted intra-articular distal radius fracture. It was treated with a locking plate and was out to length. She now has wrist pain and radiocarpal osteoarthritis.
2. A 39-year-old mechanic has a stage III SLAC wrist with constant pain. Arthroscopy shows erosion of the proximal capitate.
3. A 50-year-old woman with a stage IV SNAC wrist and severe pain.

11. **Neurovascular conditions**
    a. Thromboangiitis obliterans (TAO) or Buerger's disease
    b. Embolism
    c. Raynaud's phenomenon
    d. Ulnar hammer syndrome
    e. Pseudo-aneurysm
    f. Aneurysm
    g. Raynaud's disease
    h. Arteriovenous fistula
    i. Haemangioma

Which of the options above is best described in each of the following statements? Each option may be used once, more than once or not at all.

1. A 52-year-old smoker presents with pain and numbness in the hand. He works as a carpenter.
2. A 22-year-old girl has a 2 year history of painful hands that change colour. Laboratory tests are normal.
3. A 42-year-old woman complains about a painful left hand that changes colour. Her collagen is abnormal.

12. **Neurovascular conditions**
    a. Carpal tunnel syndrome
    b. Neurogenic thoracic outlet syndrome
    c. Disputed thoracic outlet syndrome
    d. Venous thoracic outlet syndrome
    e. Raynaud's disease
    f. Arterial thoracic outlet syndrome
    g. Takayasu's arteritis
    h. Cervical spondylosis

Which of the options above is best described in each of the following statements? Each option may be used once, more than once or not at all.

1. A 21-year-old presents with Raynaud's phenomenon and a cervical rib.
2. A 38-year-old university rower who body builds has arm and hand pain after a long rowing session.
3. A 31-year-old female nurse presents with a painful right hand with tingling. Doppler and electromyography (EMG) testing are normal.

13. **Hand deformities in rheumatoid arthritis**
    a. Metacarpophalangeal joint (MCPJ) subluxation
    b. Vaughn-Jackson syndrome
    c. Jackson Pollock syndrome
    d. Posterior interosseous nerve palsy
    e. Intrinsic deficiency
    f. Tendon subluxation
    g. Caput ulnae syndrome
    h. Mannerfelt–Norman syndrome
    i. Wartenburg syndrome

Which of the options above is best described in each of the following statements?
Each option may be used once, more than once or not at all.
    1. A 32-year-old woman with uncontrolled rheumatoid arthritis cannot extend her ring finger. Her thumb extension is also weak.
    2. A 64-year-old woman with rheumatoid arthritis cannot extend her ring finger. She has had Swanson's MCPJ replacements on the other hand.
    3. A 64-year-old woman with rheumatoid arthritis cannot actively extend her ring finger but on tenodesis testing, it extends.

14. **Tendon transfers**
    a. Zancolli's lasso procedure
    b. Flexor carpi radialis to extensor digitorum communis
    c. Pronator teres to extensor carpi radialis longus
    d. Split flexor pollicis longus to extensor pollicis longus transfer-tenodesis
    e. Brachioradialis re-routing
    f. Camitz transfer
    g. Flexor carpi ulnaris to extensor digitorum communis
    h. Extensor indicis to extensor pollicis longus

Which of the options above is best described in each of the following statements?
Each option may be used once, more than once or not at all.
    1. A 25-year old arm wrestler had a Holstein–Lewis humeral fracture and has grade 0/5 power in his wrist extensors.
    2. A 47-year-old with a Colles fracture was treated non-operatively. Three months after injury she is unable to extend her thumb.
    3. A 62-year-old man sustained an injury to his ulnar nerve at decompression of Guyon's canal. He has a claw hand.

15. **Special examinations of the hand and wrist**
    a. Distal ulnar ballottement
    b. Hueston's tabletop test
    c. Watson's shift test
    d. Tinel's test
    e. Elson's test
    f. Bunnell test
    g. Lichtman's catch-up clunk

    h. Bouvier's manoeuvre
    i. Distal radioulnar joint squeeze test
    j. Reagan's test

Which of the options above is best described in each of the following statements? Each option may be used once, more than once or not at all.

    1. This is a useful test in deciding whether or not to proceed with surgery for Dupuytren's disease.
    2. This test is good for evaluating a scapholunate advanced collapse wrist.
    3. This test will confirm intrinsic tightness.

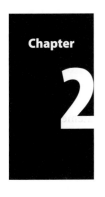

Hand and wrist: Answers

Maxim Horwitz and Elliot Sorene

MCQs

1. d. Central slip rupture.
Swan neck deformity is secondary to an imbalance between flexors and extensors with a variable contribution from the intrinsic muscles. Central slip rupture is the cause of a Boutonnière deformity.

2. d. Bone, Extensor, Flexor, Artery, Nerve, Vein.
This is a well-known order. A useful way of remembering it is **BE** a **FAN** of **V**. A stable platform is needed for reconstruction. Then the deep structures must be repaired before the delicate arterial and nerve repairs.

3. a. A2 and A4.
Any exposure of the flexor tendons in their sheath and pulley system runs the risk of disrupting a magnificent engineering wonder. The pulleys serve a very important function in creating strong lever arms for the tendons. The most important of these are the A2 and A4 pulleys. Transection results in 'bow-stringing' with subsequent weakness of flexion.

4. b. Adductor aponeurosis interposition between the distally based avulsed ligament impairs ligament healing.
In 1962 Stener described the lesion. It only occurs in complete rupture and it is thus important to clinically differentiate complete and incomplete ruptures. If the aponeurosis is interposed then complete healing of the distal fragment will not take place and despite the period of immobilization there will be excess ulnar laxity.

5. e. Up to 15° of angulation of the index and middle finger can be accepted.
Most hand surgeons would agree that there is between 15 and 30° of mobility at the carpometacarpal (CMC) joint of the ring and little fingers. This allows the surgeon to accept large amounts of deformity at the distal metacarpal neck fracture. There is still poor consensus on how much deformity to accept but 70° is still reasonable. There is consensus on the index and to a lesser degree middle finger. They do not have much compensation so 10–15° is the maximum, allowed deformity. The Jahss manoeuvre must not be confused with the Jahss position (metacarpophalangeal (MCP) and proximal interphalangeal (PIP) flexion to 90°). The manoeuvre is good, the position is no longer acceptable.

Postgraduate Orthopaedics, ed. Kesavan Sri-Ram. Published by Cambridge University Press.
© Cambridge University Press 2012.

6. **c. Extension and supination.**
This question tests the understanding of the deforming forces of a fracture. Extension and supination are necessary to overcome the pronation rotatory deformity that the volar displaced fragment undergoes.

7. **c. Triangular fibrocartilage complex (TFCC) tear.**
Once again mechanism of injury and mechanics are key to understanding the injury. Wrist pain must always be divided into radial, dorsal and ulna. Then according to the anatomy of the region, specific signs and limited special investigations a diagnosis can be made. TFCC tears are either acute or chronic and have been classified by Palmer:

    Class 1 – Traumatic

        A – central perforation or tear
        B – ulnar avulsion with or without ulnar styloid fracture
        C – distal avulsion
        D – radial avulsion with or without sigmoid notch fracture

    Class 2 – Degenerative stage

        A – TFCC wear
        B – TFCC wear with lunate and/or ulnar chondromalacia
        C – TFCC perforation with lunate and/or ulnar chondromalacia
        D – TFCC perforation with lunate and/or ulnar chondromalacia and lunotriquetral
            (LT) ligament perforation
        E – TFCC perforation with lunate and/or ulnar chondromalacia, LT ligament
            perforation, and ulnocarpal arthritis

8. **c. Perform a Henry's approach and a separate carpal tunnel incision.**
In severe wrist trauma the median nerve may be under a lot of pressure. It is not acceptable to watch and wait as there will only be more swelling post-operatively. The wrist crease must always be crossed with an S shape but in this case two separate incisions are key to prevent injury to the palmar cutaneous branch of the median nerve which lies between the flexor carpi radialis and palmaris longus. Safe surgery on the median nerve should not be contemplated from either a very radial or very ulnar approach.

9. **e. Scapholunate angle <60°.**
This question is a test of the indications for fixation of a scaphoid fracture. The unstable fracture generally needs fixation. Other signs of instability include radiolunate angle >15°, scapholunate angle >60°, intrascaphoid angles >35° and a proximal pole fracture.

10. **a. Brachioradialis and extensor carpi radialis longus (ECRL) in pronation.**
The superficial branch of the radial nerve is compressed as it is squeezed between the brachioradialis and ECRL in pronation. This must not be confused with intersection syndrome, pain associated with the crossing of the first and second dorsal extensor compartments associated with repetitive movements of the wrist (e.g. in rowers).

11. b. **Glomus tumour**.
The give away is the bluish colour under the nail. This is typical for the glomus tumour; this is a rare benign neoplasm arsing from the glomus body (a neuromyoarterial apparatus). It can be excised by lifting the nail up (if under the nail plate) with repair of the nail bed afterwards.

12. d. **Proximal injury**.
A more distal low velocity injury with a sharp object will have a better potential for healing. The long distance to the motor endplate from a proximal injury may preclude recovery. Younger patients have far higher potential for full recovery than adults.

13. d. **Natatory ligament**.
This key question is a test of anatomy. Before considering surgery a thorough knowledge of local structures is important. The distortion of the normal anatomy results in displacement of the neurovascular structures, and explains the significant risk in Dupuytren's disease surgery.

14. e. **No sensation from tip of acromion to tip of fingers**.
The prognosis for avulsion of the roots is far worse than just rupture or traction. All of these markers suggest severe trauma and may point to root avulsion. Numbness on its own is not as worrying as the other signs.

15. c. **Tendon pull must be synergistic**.
These rules must be appreciated and short cuts will only lead to disaster. Donor muscles must be expendable and have adequate power, ideally MRC grade 5. Joints must be mobile with no contracture.

16. e. **Diabetic cheirarthropathy**.
This is a poorly understood condition. It is thought to be as a result of a muscular or tendon imbalance with soft tissue disruption. There is a microangiopathy of the dermal and subcutaneous blood vessels. It is more common in Type 1 diabetics and can affect 8–50% of the population. Loss of function is painless, and progresses from distal to proximal. The prayer sign is an inability to oppose palmar surfaces.

17. e. **Wrist arthrodesis**.
The Lichtman classification system essentially divides Kienbock's disease into types that can be treated with therapeutic operations such as radial shortening or grafting versus those that need salvage operations such as partial or complete wrist arthrodesis. One of the deciding factors in the type of fusion is the degree of fixed deformity. In the presence of fixed deformity radial shortening is not an option. It is also not an option in the more uncommon scenario of the ulnar positive wrist. The Lichtman classification, based on radiographs, is as follows:

Stage 1 – normal (may have a linear or a compression fracture)
Stage 2 – sclerosis but no collapse
Stage 3A – collapse of entire lunate without fixed scaphoid rotation
Stage 3B – collapse of entire lunate with fixed scaphoid rotation
Stage 4 – stage III with generalized degenerative changes in the carpus

18. a. Ulnar shortening osteotomy.
It is uncommon for younger people to present with significant radial shortening as their fractures are usually well managed. In this case there is ulna impaction syndrome. The aim is to reduce this impaction. There is no need to address the DRUJ or replace the distal ulna. The Darrach procedure should be reserved for older patients with rheumatoid disease. It is associated with ongoing discomfort in the proximal stump and certainly not the first choice in this scenario.

19. b. Painful nodules are an indication for surgery.
The disease is usually in its early phases. The stages, according to Luck's classification, are proliferative, involutional and finally residual. Early surgery will certainly lead to recurrence and can stimulate the disease process. Carpal tunnel surgery must be performed at a separate occasion for a similar reason. Unfortunately in the long term recurrence rates are high (50%).

20. d. Class 1B lesion.
TFCC tears are divided into acute (1) and chronic (2) by the Palmer classification. The majority of isolated TFCC injuries do not require early surgical management. The need for treatment is increased when the lesion is associated with fractures, instability and DRUJ injuries.

21. b. She has a claw hand.
She has tight intrinsic muscles and her Bunnell test is positive as the intrinsic muscles are more powerful than her extrinsic extensors and flexors. The tight intrinsic muscles are treated with distal releases when fibrotic and a proximal slide when spastic. An intrinsic minus hand is one where there is a loss of function in the ulna and sometimes the median nerve (claw). The patient presents with a monkey grip.

22. c. Quadrigia effect.
Though this was a bony avulsion it must be thought of like any other FDP tendon injury. In this case because of the proximal migration of the tendon it was probably repaired tightly with an adhesed improperly tensioned FDP. Because the adjacent remaining fingers share a common muscle belly, they cannot flex entirely (quadrigia effect).

23. a. There is not always a scaphoid fracture.
To understand carpal instability it is essential to appreciate the ligamentous attachments both between the individual carpal bones as well as the extrinsic ligaments that support the wrist. The Mayfield staging is thus summarized:

Stage I – scapholunate dissociation/scaphoid fracture
Stage II – lunocapitate dislocation
Stage III – lunotriquetral disruption/triquetrum fracture
Stage IV – lunate dislocation

24. d. Superficial palmar arch.
The superficial palmar arch is a continuation of the ulna artery. In the majority of patients (78%) this arch is completed by branches from the deep palmar, radial or median arteries. This explains why even with significant lacerations to the ulna artery a hand can be well perfused.

25. c. **Mucoid cyst.**
This is a common lesion that arises from the osteoarthritic DIP joint. There is usually a disruption of the joint and a cyst develops. They cause deformity of the nail because of pressure on the germinal matrix. If they are large it may be necessary to perform a local flap at excision (transposition).

26. a. **Nerve stimulation therapy.**
If symptoms are not severe and there is not significant and progressive neuropathy then non-operative management must be considered. This includes splintage, hand therapy, steroid injection and even yoga has been proven to be beneficial. Alternatively a patient could be referred for either open or endoscopic release.

27. c. **Scaphoid extension.**
In rheumatoid arthritis the inflammation of the synovium sets off a sequence of events that start with correctable deformity and eventually lead to fixed deformity and destruction of the joints. The synovitis at the DRUJ leads to capsular stretching with ECU subluxation and stretching of the dorsal structures. There is erosion of the radio-scapho-capitate ligament with flexion of the scaphoid. The carpus supinates as it moves in an ulna direction. Rather than the ulna becoming prominent it is the carpus that slips away from it.

28. e. **Nail patella syndrome.**
This syndrome is a result of an abnormality on chromosome 9. Patients may have subluxed or dislocated radial heads and never realize they have a problem until they have an X-ray. The syndrome can include abnormalities of the patella and nail growth, generalized ligamentous laxity and bony exostoses.

29. d. **50%.**
Because of the morbidity and prolonged rehabilitation associated with tendon repair it is advisable to repair lacerations over 50% of the tendon width. The exception to this rule is if there is visible triggering under a local anaesthetic block it may be necessary to address this.

30. b. **Sonic hedgehog protein.**
Eight weeks after fertilization, all limb structures are present. It is between 4 and 8 weeks where the majority of congenital disorders in the hand occur. There are many factors involved in limb development; however, there are three key zones responsible for proximodistal, anteroposterior and dorsoventral development. These are the apical ectodermal ridge, zone of polarizing activity and Wnt pathway respectively. These in turn produce fibroblast growth factors, sonic hedgehog protein and LMX1, which all work in a coordinated manner to ensure the normal development of the limb.

EMQs

1. 1. **c. Extensor carpi ulnaris (ECU) subluxation and tenosynovitis.**
   2. **f. Vaughn–Jackson syndrome.** 3. **a. De Quervain's disease.**
This question is really a test of the seven extensor compartments. Each compartment has its own unique anatomy and pathology in turn. Rowers and drummers have ECU subluxation and tenosynovitis. It is common for young mothers to develop tenosynovitis of the first extensor compartment but the condition is not exclusive to them. Vaughn-Jackson syndrome is the attritional rupture of the extensor digiti minimi (EDM) in rheumatoid arthritis. The compartments are as follows:

  First – abductor pollicis longus and extensor pollicis brevis tendons
  Second – extensor carpi radialis longus and extensor carpi radialis brevis tendons
  Third – extensor pollicis longus tendon
  Fourth – three tendons of extensor digitorum muscle and the extensor indicis tendon
  Fifth – extensor digiti minimi tendon
  Sixth – extensor carpi ulnaris

2. 1. **g.** *Eikenella corrodens.* 2. **d. Herpes simplex virus type 1.** 3. **h.** *Pasteurella multocida.*
The most common cause of hand infections is probably still *Staphylococcus aureus.* However, because the hands come into contact with specific things it is important to recognize a few important infections. A 'fight bite' often presents with a small wound and a history of punching. *Eikenella corrodens* comes from the human mouth. Dentists and healthcare workers are exposed to the herpes virus. The typical organism in cat bites is *Pasteurella.* The organisms in necrotizing fasciitis are multiple and usually include clostridia and Group A β-streptococci.

3. 1. **f. V-Y plasty (advancement).** 2. **a. Cross finger flap.** 3. **c. Terminalization.**
Knowing the plastic surgery reconstructive ladder is essential for the management of fingertip injuries. The principle is that if the wound is <1 cm and if there is no bone exposed it can probably heal on its own or be covered with skin only. If there is a bigger lesion with exposed bone then the type of lesion and location must be carefully assessed.

4. 1. **c. Epithelioid.** 2. **g. Enchondroma.** 3. **e. Schwannoma.**
Sarcoma and other malignancies in the hands are rare. Benign tumours and skin cancers are not. Prior to and after the excision of any lesion from the hand the surgeon must have a wide differential diagnosis at hand.

5. 1. **f. Psoriasis.** 2. **b. Scleroderma.** 3. **e. Amyloidosis.**
Many systemic conditions manifest in a pathognomonic manner in the hands. Certain key facts have been provided about each of the conditions. The reader is reminded that other arthritides must be considered in hand pathology.

6. 1. **a. Parsonage–Turner syndrome.** 2. **e. Anterior interosseous nerve palsy.**
   3. **h. Mannerfelt–Norman syndrome.**
The various compression neuropathies can be a bit tricky. The key to the anterior interosseous nerve is that it is a pure motor palsy. Pronator syndrome is a sensory deficit. Mannerfelt–Norman syndrome refers to an attrition rupture of the flexor pollicis longus

due to scaphotrapezial synovitis. This question could also be asked in terms of special investigations and special tests in clinical examination.

7. 1. **d. Radial shortening**. 2. **e. Proximal row carpectomy**. 3. **a. Wrist fusion**.
The clues of dorsal wrist pain and Lichtman classification lead the reader to Kienbock's disease. The question is a discriminator between treatment and salvage of the disease as well as differentiating fixed and mobile deformity (3A vs. 3B).

8. 1. **a. Intrinsic plus hand**. 2. **f. Quadrigia effect**. 3. **b. Boutonnière deformity**.
This questions tests knowledge of special signs. Intrinsic tightness as shown by the Bunell test must be differentiated from the intrinsic minus hand, e.g. loss of ulnar nerve function. A Boutonnière deformity is usually due to central slip rupture while a swan neck deformity can have many causes.

9. 1. **b. Hamate hook fracture**. 2. **g. Ulnocarpal abutment**. 3. **k. Scaphoid lunate advanced collapse**.
When evaluating wrist pain it is worth dividing it into dorsal, radial and ulnar-sided wrist pain. Once age and location has been taken into account the diagnosis will be narrowed down. At this stage radiographs and diagnostic injections will probably provide a definite answer. The ring sign is one of many signs that reveal widening of the scapholunate ligament and flexion of the scaphoid.

10. 1. **b. Radio-scapholunate fusion**. 2. **c. Scaphoidectomy and four-corner fusion**. 3. **a. Wrist fusion with AO fusion plate**.
The aim of this question is to differentiate localized arthritis of the wrist (requiring limited arthrodesis) from pan-arthritis (requiring full fusion). Because of the capitate erosion a proximal row carpectomy is not an option and the four-corner fusion is the correct choice. In a stage IV wrist, full wrist arthrodesis is the only option.

11. 1. **d. Ulnar hammer syndrome**. 2. **g. Raynaud's disease**. 3. **c. Raynaud's phenomenon**.
The key to this question is the ability to differentiate Raynaud's phenomenon from disease. Disease mainly affects females over a chronic period with normal lab tests. The phenomenon is a consequence of either vaso-spastic or vaso-occlusive disease. The ulnar hammer syndrome with thrombosis of the ulnar artery occurs more commonly in males around the age of 55 who smoke, and who use their hand as a hammer. The carpenter fact and the cold sensitivity are the clues.

12. 1. **f. Arterial thoracic outlet syndrome**. 2. **d. Venous thoracic outlet syndrome**. 3. **c. Disputed thoracic outlet syndrome**.
Thoracic outlet syndrome is a rare condition with 95% being the disputed type with normal special tests. Cervical ribs and true arterial occlusion (i.e. secondary Raynaud's phenomenon) is a rare cause. Muscular men tend to get venous occlusion. True neurogenic thoracic outlet syndrome is very rare secondary to nerve compression at C8/T1.

13. 1. **d. Posterior interosseous nerve palsy**. 2. **a. Metacarpophalangeal joint (MCPJ) subluxation**. 3. **f. Tendon subluxation**.
There are four reasons for a loss of finger extension in rheumatoid arthritis. In simple tendon rupture (Vaughn-Jackson syndrome vs. Jackson Pollock, who is an abstract artist)

the tenodesis test will be negative. In subluxation, tenodesis test is positive. If there is a lot of inflammation at the elbow then the posterior interosseous nerve will be compromised, hence the widespread weakness involving the thumb. Lastly, MCPJ misalignment will create a problem with the pull of the tendon and hence a loss of extension. Intrinsic musculature is usually tight, not deficient.

14. 1. **c. Pronator teres to extensor carpi radialis longus.** 2. **h. Extensor indicis to extensor pollicis longus.** 3. **a. Zancolli's lasso procedure.**
There are many classic and other more creative tendon transfers. It is important to know at least two transfers for each of the major upper limb nerves and understand the principles of tendon transfer. It is the rare attritional rupture of the extensor pollicis longus tendon on Lister's tubercle that occurs in non-operatively treated fractures. The split flexor pollicis longus to extensor pollicis longus transfer-tenodesis is reserved for more complex reconstruction of pinch, in intrinsic deficiency.

15. 1. **b. Hueston's tabletop test.** 2. **c. Watson's shift test.** 3. **f. Bunnell test.**
Special tests must not only be applied to each lesion but the reader must have an understanding of the mechanism for each test. These are but a few of the more common ones and it is recommended that they are all performed even on the normal hand to get into the habit of performing these sometimes difficult tests.

Selected references

Clayton ML. Historical perspectives on surgery of the rheumatoid hand. *Hand Clin* 1989; 5: 111–14.

Green DP. *Green's Operative Hand Surgery*, 5th edn. Philadelphia, Elsevier, 2005.

Jebson PJ, Kasdan ML. *Hand Secrets*, 3rd edn. Philadelphia, Hanley and Balfus, 2006.

Kapoor A, Sibbitt WL Jr. Contractures in diabetes mellitus: the syndrome of limited joint mobility. *Semin Arthritis Rheum* 1989; 18(3): 168–80.

Kienbock R., Peltier L. Concerning traumatic malacia of the lunate and its consequences: degeneration and compression fractures. *Clin Orthop* 1980; 149: 4–8.

McRae R. *Orthopaedics and Fractures*, 2nd edn. London, Churchill Livingstone, 2006.

Miller MD. *Review of Orthopaedics*, 5th edn. Philadelphia, Elsevier, 2008.

Nagle DJ. Evaluation of chronic wrist pain. *J Am Acad Orthop Surg* 2000; 8: 45–55.

Stanley J. Mini-Symposium: Rheumatoid Disease of the Hand and Wrist, Degenerative arthritis of the wrist. *Curr Orthop* 1999; 13(4): 290–6.

Stanley J. Mini-Symposium: Rheumatoid Disease of the Hand and Wrist, The rheumatoid wrist. *Curr Orthop* 2001; 15(5): 329–37.

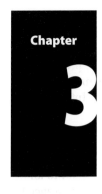

Chapter

3

Shoulder and elbow: Questions

Deborah S. Higgs and Simon Lambert

MCQs

1. The term internal impingement is used in throwers to describe a condition where the posterosuperior glenoid labrum impinges on which structure?
   a. The anterior glenohumeral ligaments.
   b. The posterior glenohumeral ligaments.
   c. The biceps tendon.
   d. The anterior rotator cuff.
   e. The posterior rotator cuff.

2. The biomechanical advantage of a reverse total shoulder arthroplasty compared to a standard arthroplasty is what?
   a. Centre of rotation more superior.
   b. Centre of rotation more medial.
   c. Centre of rotation more lateral.
   d. Increased lateral humeral offset.
   e. Decreased deltoid muscle fibre tension.

3. Posterior glenohumeral dislocations occur more frequently than anterior dislocations in which group of patients?
   a. Rugby players.
   b. Ehlers–Danlos patients.
   c. Hypermobile patients.
   d. Epileptics.
   e. None of the above.

4. A football player sustains a suspected acromioclavicular joint (ACJ) separation. Which of the following is the most appropriate radiographic view to evaluate the ACJ?
   a. Stryker notch view.
   b. Serendipity view.
   c. Zanca view.
   d. Supraspinatus outlet view.
   e. Garth view.

Postgraduate Orthopaedics, ed. Kesavan Sri-Ram. Published by Cambridge University Press.
© Cambridge University Press 2012.

5. **When compared to the non-dominant side, which of the following shoulder motions is characteristically decreased in the throwing arm of athletes?**
   a. Internal rotation (IR).
   b. External rotation (ER).
   c. Forward elevation.
   d. Abduction.
   e. Adduction.

6. **Which of the following muscles have only a single nerve supply?**
   a. Brachialis.
   b. Flexor digitorum profundus.
   c. Lumbricals.
   d. Brachioradialis.
   e. Pectoralis major.

7. **With the arm in 90° of abduction, which of the following is considered the primary static restraint to anterior glenohumeral translation?**
   a. Negative intra-articular pressure.
   b. Superior glenohumeral ligament complex.
   c. Middle glenohumeral ligament complex.
   d. Inferior glenohumeral ligament complex.
   e. Shape of the bony articulation.

8. **Following a traumatic anterior shoulder dislocation, what factor is associated with the highest risk for recurrent instability?**
   a. Dislocation of the dominant shoulder.
   b. Bilateral shoulder dislocation.
   c. Young age (<25 years old) at time of dislocation.
   d. Family history of shoulder instability.
   e. Joint laxity.

9. **Which of the following is a known risk factor for the development of adhesive capsulitis of the shoulder?**
   a. Epilepsy.
   b. Dupuytren's contracture.
   c. Diabetes mellitus.
   d. Renal disease.
   e. All of the above.

10. **Injury to the long thoracic nerve can present clinically as which of the following?**
    a. Weak shoulder abduction.
    b. Trapezius palsy.
    c. Latissimus dorsi atrophy.
    d. Lateral scapular winging.
    e. Medial scapular winging.

11. **Which of the following best describes a Buford complex?**
    a. Normal anatomic variant characterized by a cord-like middle glenohumeral ligament (MGHL) and an absent anteroinferior labrum.
    b. Normal anatomic variant characterized by a cord-like MGHL and an absent anterosuperior labrum.
    c. Normal anatomic variant characterized by a cord-like superior glenohumeral ligament (SGHL) and an absent anterosuperior labrum.
    d. Abnormal finding characterized by a cord-like MGHL and an absent anterosuperior labrum.
    e. Abnormal finding characterized by a cord-like inferior glenohumeral ligament (IGHL) and an absent posteroinferior labrum.

12. **Following a total shoulder arthroplasty through a deltopectoral approach, motion and strengthening are typically initially restricted because of which factor?**
    a. Risk of dislocation.
    b. Risk of loosening.
    c. Risk of glenoid fracture.
    d. Protect the subscapularis tendon.
    e. Protect the supraspinatus tendon.

13. **In an anterior dislocation which nerve is most likely to be injured?**
    a. Musculocutaneous.
    b. Suprascapular.
    c. Upper or lower subscapular.
    d. Axillary.
    e. Radial.

14. **A 55-year-old patient has chronic pain over the lateral aspect of the elbow, exacerbated when playing backhand tennis stroke. On examination she has pain with resisted middle finger extension. Which muscle attachment is most likely involved?**
    a. Brachioradialis.
    b. Extensor digitorum communis.
    c. Extensor carpi radialis longus.
    d. Extensor carpi radialis brevis.
    e. Anconeus.

15. **Which of the following is the primary stabilizer to resist valgus stress in the flexed elbow?**
    a. Ulno-humeral articulation.
    b. Radiocapitellar articulation.
    c. Flexor-pronator muscle mass.
    d. Anterior band of the medial ulnar collateral ligament.
    e. Posterior band of the medial ulnar collateral ligament.

16. **The greatest stress on the medial ulnar collateral ligament of the elbow occurs during which phase of throwing?**
    a. Wind-up.
    b. Early cocking.

   c. Late cocking.

   d. Ball release.

   e. Follow through.

17. A 31-year-old weightlifter reports right shoulder pain with cross-body adduction as well as point tenderness at the acromioclavicular joint (ACJ). X-rays show osteopaenia of the distal clavicle. Initial treatment should include?
   a. Glenohumeral joint injection.
   b. Periscapular muscle strengthening.
   c. Activity modification.
   d. Capsular release.
   e. Arthroscopic resection of the distal clavicle.

18. Avulsion of which ligament off its humeral insertion has historically been associated with recurrent instability and may require open repair?
   a. Inferior glenohumeral.
   b. Middle glenohumeral.
   c. Superior glenohumeral.
   d. Coracohumeral.
   e. Coracoacromial.

19. A 78-year old female sustains a four-part proximal humerus fracture and undergoes a shoulder hemiarthroplasty. Intraoperatively the lesser tuberosity was lateralized. What problem will this patient most likely have post-operatively?
   a. Forward elevation weakness.
   b. Bicipital pain.
   c. Abduction deficit.
   d. External rotation deficit.
   e. Internal rotation deficit.

20. A patient is known to have a SLAP tear. An MRI shows a large cyst in the spinoglenoid notch. What additional finding on examination is the patient likely to display?
   a. Weakness in external rotation.
   b. Weakness in forward elevation.
   c. Weakness in internal rotation.
   d. Medial scapular winging.
   e. Lateral scapular winging.

21. What technical error leads to scapular notching after reverse total shoulder arthroplasty?
   a. Retroverted placement of the glenoid component.
   b. Superior placement of the glenoid component.
   c. Inferior placement of the glenoid component.
   d. Posterior placement of the glenoid component.
   e. Overtensioning of the soft tissue envelope.

22. **What is the most common pathological arthroscopic finding following a traumatic anterior shoulder dislocation?**
    a. Hill–Sachs lesion.
    b. Posterosuperior labral tear.
    c. Posteroinferior labral tear.
    d. Anterosuperior labral tear.
    e. Anteroinferior labral tear.

23. **When approaching the proximal diaphyseal radius via the Henry approach (volar), the forearm is supinated to minimize injury to what structure?**
    a. Radial nerve.
    b. Lateral antebrachial cutaneous nerve.
    c. Posterior interosseous nerve.
    d. Ulnar nerve.
    e. Median nerve.

24. **A patient sustains a midshaft clavicle fracture which heals with 2 cm of shortening. What is the most likely clinical outcome?**
    a. Normal shoulder muscle strength and endurance.
    b. Decreased shoulder muscle strength and endurance.
    c. Decreased shoulder abduction.
    d. Decreased shoulder external rotation.
    e. Decreased shoulder adduction.

25. **A 68-year-old female rheumatoid patient presents with a painful, stiff elbow. Plain radiographs show a Larsen grade IV. The most appropriate surgical option is?**
    a. Arthroscopic synovectomy.
    b. Open synovectomy.
    c. Open synovectomy and radial head excision.
    d. Lateral elbow replacement.
    e. Total elbow replacement.

26. **A 50-year-old male complains of acute shoulder pain and an inability to lift his arm over his head after an anterior shoulder dislocation. Examination reveals active forward elevation to 30° and grade 3/5 external rotation strength. An arthrogram shows extravasation of the dye into the subacromial space with no evidence of arthritis. What is the most appropriate treatment option?**
    a. Shoulder hemiarthroplasty.
    b. Rotator cuff repair.
    c. Reverse total shoulder arthroplasty.
    d. Total shoulder arthroplasty.
    e. Physiotherapy.

27. **A 35-year-old woman sustains an elbow fracture dislocation which includes a coronoid fracture involving more than 50%, and a comminuted radial head fracture. What is the most appropriate treatment?**
    a. Closed reduction and early range of motion.
    b. Radial head resection and coronoid open reduction internal fixation.

   c. Radial head arthroplasty and coronoid open reduction internal fixation.

   d. Radial head resection and lateral collateral ligament reconstruction.

   e. Radial head arthroplasty, coronoid open reduction internal fixation and lateral collateral ligament repair.

28. **What is the most common mode of failure of the lateral ulnar collateral ligament (LUCL) associated with an elbow dislocation?**
   a. Ligament avulsion off the humeral origin.
   b. Ligament avulsion off the ulnar insertion.
   c. Bony avulsion of the humeral origin.
   d. Bony avulsion of the ulnar insertion.
   e. Midsubstance rupture.

29. **A patient sustains a displaced scapular neck fracture. What is the internervous plane for a posterior approach to the glenohumeral joint?**
   a. Suprascapular-axillary.
   b. Suprascapular-subscapular.
   c. Long thoracic-spinal accessory.
   d. Lateral pectoral-axillary.
   e. Subscapular-musculocutaneous.

30. **The optimal position of the shoulder for arthrodesis is?**
   a. External rotation (ER) 30°, Flexion 30°, Abduction 30°.
   b. ER 30°, Flexion 30°, Adduction 30°.
   c. Internal rotation (IR) 30°, Flexion 30°, Abduction 30°.
   d. IR 30°, Flexion 10°, Adduction 30°.
   e. IR 30°, Flexion 40°, Abduction 30°.

EMQs

1. **Nerves in the arm**
   a. Anterior interosseous nerve
   b. Spinal accessory nerve
   c. Long thoracic nerve
   d. Axillary nerve
   e. Median nerve
   f. Musculocutaneous nerve
   g. Radial nerve
   h. Ulnar nerve

Which of the options above is best described in each of the following statements?
Each option may be used once, more than once or not at all.
   1. Damage to this nerve can result in lateral scapular winging.
   2. This is a supraclavicular branch of the brachial plexus.
   3. This is the nerve most at risk during placement of the anterolateral portal in elbow arthroscopy.

2. **Structures around the shoulder**
   a. Glenoid labrum
   b. Superior glenohumeral ligament (SGHL)
   c. Middle glenohumeral ligament (MGHL)
   d. Anterior band of the inferior glenohumeral ligament (IGHL)
   e. Posterior band of the inferior glenohumeral ligament (IGHL)
   f. Coracohumeral ligament (CHL)
   g. Infraspinatus
   h. Subscapularis

Which of the options above is best described in each of the following statements?
Each option may be used once, more than once or not at all.
   1. This is highly variable and poorly defined in up to 40% of the population.
   2. This is the primary restraint to anterior/inferior translation of the head with the shoulder abducted to 90° and in maximum external rotation.
   3. With the shoulder in external rotation, this is an important dynamic stabilizer to posterior subluxation.

3. **Radiographic views**
   a. Supraspinatus outlet view
   b. True anteroposterior (AP)
   c. AP in internal rotation (IR)
   d. Zanca view
   e. Axillary view
   f. Serendipity view
   g. Stryker notch view
   h. Garth view

Which of the options above is best described in each of the following statements? Each option may be used once, more than once or not at all.
1. This is used to assess anteroposterior dislocations of the sternoclavicular joint.
2. This is used to assess acromion morphology.
3. This is used to assess for Hill–Sachs defect and taken with the patient supine with the palm of the hand of the affected extremity placed on top of the head with the fingers toward the back of the head.

4. **Elbow conditions**
   a. Lateral epicondylitis
   b. Medial epicondylitis
   c. Radiocapitellar osteoarthritis
   d. Posterolateral rotatory instability
   e. Lateral impingement
   f. Posterior interosseous syndrome
   g. Valgus instability
   h. Radial tunnel syndrome

Which of the options above is best described in each of the following statements? Each option may be used once, more than once or not at all.
1. A 45-year-old patient complains of chronic lateral elbow pain. On examination pain is exacerbated by resisted forearm pronation and wrist flexion.
2. A 48-year-old complains of chronic lateral elbow pain. On examination there is weakness and ulnar drift with wrist extension.
3. A 42-year-old undergoes surgery for tennis elbow. Following surgery, she describes clicking and popping on the lateral aspect of the elbow. Examination reveals a positive lateral pivot shift.

5. **Structures around the elbow**
   a. Lateral collateral ligament
   b. Lateral ulnar collateral ligament
   c. Medial collateral ligament
   d. Radial collateral ligament
   e. Annular ligament
   f. Posterolateral capsule
   g. Anterior capsule
   h. Ulnar collateral ligament

Which of the options above is best described in each of the following statements? Each option may be used once, more than once or not at all.
1. This is typically the first ligament disrupted in an elbow dislocation.
2. Disruption of this structure is the essential lesion responsible for posterolateral rotatory instability of the elbow.
3. Valgus stability with the arm in pronation suggests this structure is intact.

6. **Painful shoulder**
   a. Subacromial impingement
   b. Suprascapular nerve entrapment

   c. Parsonage–Turner syndrome
   d. Thoracic outlet syndrome
   e. Acromioclavicular arthritis
   f. Supraspinatus calcific tendinitis
   g. Subcoracoid impingement
   h. SLAP lesion
   i. Adhesive capsulitis

Which of the options above is best described in each of the following statements?
Each option may be used once, more than once or not at all.

1. A 45-year-old diabetic presents with acute onset shoulder pain, constant in nature affecting sleep. Shoulder examination reveals limited active and passive movement, especially external rotation. Plain radiograph is unremarkable.
2. A 35-year-old patient complains of anterior shoulder pain exacerbated by positioning the arm in adduction, forward flexion and an internally rotated position. A CT scan shows a coracohumeral distance of 5 mm.
3. A 40-year-old patient with a clavicle malunion complains of tingling and numbness in her fingers mostly in the ring and small finger, made worse with overhead activity. Examination includes a positive Wright test.

7. Treatment for shoulder pathology

   a. Eccentric deltoid physiotherapy programme
   b. Arthroscopic capsular release
   c. Subscapularis repair
   d. Supraspinatus repair
   e. Arthroscopic subacromial decompression
   f. Hemiarthroplasty
   g. Latissimus dorsi tendon transfer
   h. Unconstrained total shoulder arthroplasty
   i. Reverse type total shoulder arthroplasty

Which of the options above is best described in each of the following statements?
Each option may be used once, more than once or not at all.

1. A 62-year old man undergoes a total shoulder arthroplasty for osteoarthritis. He accidently uses his operative arm to rise from a chair 3 weeks after surgery and thereafter complains of anterior shoulder pain. Radiographs show anterior subluxation of the prosthesis.
2. A 70-year-old patient with rheumatoid arthritis with a symptomatic arthritic cuff deficient shoulder.
3. A 55-year-old man has an unrepairable posterosuperior rotator cuff tear. He has full passive range of movement but limited active movement. Clinically he has an intact subscapularis. X-rays show a centred humeral head with no degenerative change.

8. Surgical approaches

   a. Deltopectoral approach
   b. Henry approach
   c. Thompson approach
   d. Kocher approach

e. Anterior approach to the elbow
f. Posterior approach to the shoulder
g. Lateral approach to the shoulder
h. Kaplan approach

Which of the options above is best described in each of the following statements? Each option may be used once, more than once or not at all.
1. This uses the internervous plane between the suprascapular nerve and the axillary nerve.
2. This is the approach of choice for open reduction and internal fixation (ORIF) of a glenoid neck fracture.
3. This does not utilize an internervous plane.

9. Special tests during shoulder examination
a. Impingement injection test
b. Lift-off test
c. Hawkin's sign
d. Load-and-shift test
e. Cross body adduction
f. O'Briens test
g. Speed's test
h. Hornblower's sign
i. External rotation lag sign
j. Belly press

Which of the options above is best described in each of the following statements? Each option may be used once, more than once or not at all.
1. When assessing subscapularis, this is more accurate for assessing the superior portion.
2. Tests the integrity of teres minor.
3. This tests for impingement by forcibly internally rotating the shoulder, driving the greater tuberosity further under the coracoacromial ligament.

10. Shoulder pathology
a. Biceps tear
b. Bankart lesion
c. Pectoralis major rupture
d. Spinoglenoid cyst
e. Superior labrum anterior and posterior tear
f. Adhesive capsulitis
g. Humeral avulsion of the glenohumeral ligament (HAGL) lesion
h. Subscapularis rupture
i. Glenohumeral osteoarthritis

Which of the options above is best described in each of the following statements? Each option may be used once, more than once or not at all.
1. A 36-year-old patient reports a sharp tearing sensation whilst bench-pressing. He subsequently develops bruising over the upper arm and weakness in adduction and internal rotation.

2. An 18-year-old rugby player underwent surgery to repair a Bankart lesion for traumatic instability. Twelve months post-surgery, examination reveals stability, external rotation to 0° with the elbow at his side and to 40° at 90° of abduction. If his range of motion does not improve, he is at most risk of?

3. A 34-year-old man underwent an open Bankart repair with capsulorrhaphy for recurrent anterior instability 6 months ago. In a recent fall, he describes a hyperabduction, external rotation injury. He now has anterior shoulder pain and the sensation of instability. Examination reveals a positive lift-off test and external rotation is 15° greater than the opposite side.

11. Arthroscopic findings in the shoulder
a. SLAP type I
b. SLAP type II
c. SLAP type III
d. SLAP type IV
e. Rotator cuff articular side tear
f. Biceps tendon fraying
g Peel-back lesion
h. Anterior labral periasteal sleeve avulsion (ALPSA) lesion
i. Biceps tendon subluxation

Which of the options above is best described in each of the following statements? Each option may be used once, more than once or not at all.
1. The most common clinically significant type of SLAP lesion identified at arthroscopy.
2. Describes a bucket handle tear of the labrum with a longitudinal tear extending into the biceps.
3. Identifying this pathology at arthroscopy should raise the suspicion of a subscapularis tear.

12. Treatment of shoulder injuries
a. Collar and cuff
b. Manipulation under anaesthesia (MUA)
c. MUA and percutaneous K-wire fixation
d. Open reduction and internal fixation (ORIF)
e. ORIF and bone grafting
f. Hemiarthroplasty
g. Shoulder resurfacing
h. Unconstrained total shoulder replacement
i. Reverse total shoulder replacement

Which of the options above is best described in each of the following statements? Each option may be used once, more than once or not at all.
1. Two-part proximal humerus fracture with 6 mm displacement of the greater tuberosity fragment.
2. Four-part head splitting proximal humerus fracture in a 55-year-old.
3. Four-part valgus impacted proximal humerus fracture in a 45-year-old.

13. **Anatomical spaces**
    a. Triangular space
    b. Triangular interval
    c. Quadrangular space
    d. Cubital tunnel
    e. Suprascapular space
    f. Spinoglenoid notch
    g. Radial tunnel
    h. Subcoracoid space

Which of the options above is best described in each of the following statements?
Each option may be used once, more than once or not at all.
    1. This contains the profunda brachii artery.
    2. This is immediately inferior to the quadrangular space.
    3. Its lateral border is the long head of triceps.

14. **Treatment of elbow injuries**
    a. Initial splintage, followed by range-of-motion exercises
    b. Aspiration of the haemarthrosis, followed by active range-of-motion exercises
    c. Fragment excision
    d. Open reduction and internal fixation (ORIF)
    e. Radial head replacement
    f. Radial head excision
    g. Lateral elbow replacement
    h. Cubital tunnel release
    i. Lateral ligament reconstruction
    j. Medial ligament reconstruction
    k. Medial ligament repair

Which of the options above is best described in each of the following statements?
Each option may be used once, more than once or not at all.
    1. A 25-year-old builder sustains a 3 mm displaced Mason type II radial head fracture. Examination reveals pain and catching that limits his range of motion to 45° of supination and 20° of pronation.
    2. A 32-year-old patient presents with an unreconstructable Mason type III radial head fracture. A lateral radiograph of the wrist shows a dorsally subluxed ulna.
    3. A 19-year-old javelin thrower presents with posteromedial elbow pain and complains that his throwing distance has reduced. He also complains of paraesthesia in the ring and little finger.

15. **Paediatric elbow**
    a. Capitellum
    b. Medial epicondyle
    c. Radial head
    d. Lateral epicondyle
    e. Lateral condyle
    f. Medial condyle

g. Trochlea
h. Coronoid
i. Olecranon

Which of the options above is best described in each of the following statements?
Each option may be used once, more than once or not at all.
1. Non-union of which can result in tardy ulnar nerve palsy.
2. Can be affected by osteochondritis dissecans.
3. Ossifies at around the age of 8 years.

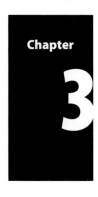

Shoulder and elbow: Answers

Deborah S. Higgs and Simon Lambert

MCQs

1. e. The posterior rotator cuff.
The primary cause of internal impingement is often anterior capsular laxity, which may result in posterior capsular tightness. This results in anterior shift of the axis of rotation of the humeral head in the sagittal plane, when the arm is in an abducted, externally rotated position, causing the posterior rotator cuff to impinge against the posterosuperior glenoid labrum. Examination may reveal a loss of >20° of internal rotation at 90º. Treatment is directed at posterior capsule stretching. Internal impingement is implicated in the development of articular sided rotator cuffs and posterosuperior labral tears.

2. b. Centre of rotation more medial.
The advantage of a reverse shoulder arthroplasty is that the centre of rotation (COR) is medialized, which decreases the forces at the implant–bone interface and provides a mechanical advantage to the deltoid muscle to substitute for the deficient rotator cuff muscles to provide shoulder abduction.

3. e. None of the above.
Whilst traumatic posterior shoulder dislocations are associated with epilepsy, they are not more common in this patient group than traumatic anterior dislocations.

4. c. Zanca view.
Anteroposterior (AP), lateral and axial views are standard views taken for the shoulder; however, a Zanca view is the most accurate view to look at the ACJ. This view is performed by tilting the X-ray beam 10° to 15° toward the cephalic direction and using only 50% of the standard shoulder AP penetration strength. In a standard AP view of the shoulder, the ACJ will be over-penetrated (dark) and small or subtle lesions may be overlooked.

5. a. Internal rotation (IR).
Glenohumeral internal rotation deficit (GIRD) is associated with throwing athletes. Repetitive throwing (cocking phase and deceleration phase) leads to a tight posterior capsule and loose anterior capsule. It is associated with internal impingement. On examination the full arc of rotation at 90° is maintained but excessive ER is present at the expense of decreased IR (loss of >20° of IR at 90° compared to contralateral side). Treatment consists of posterior capsule stretching.

Postgraduate Orthopaedics, ed. Kesavan Sri-Ram. Published by Cambridge University Press.
© Cambridge University Press 2012.

6. d. **Brachioradialis**.
Many muscle groups in the upper limb have dual innervation. Brachialis (musculocutaneous and radial), flexor digitorum profundus (anterior interosseus and ulna), lumbricals (recurrent median and ulna) and pectoralis major (lateral pectoral and medial pectoral) are examples.

7. d. **Inferior glenohumeral ligament complex**.
The rotator cuff is a dynamic stabilizer and the capsulolabral tissues are considered static stabilizers. With the arm at 90° abduction, the anterior band of the inferior glenohumeral ligament complex is the primary static stabilizer to anterior translation.

8. c. **Young age (<25 years old) at time of dislocation**.
The only consistent predictor of recurrence has been the age of the patient. In young patients (<25 years old), recurrence rates have ranged from 60% to 94%. Family history confers a 34% risk of recurrence, while dislocation in the contralateral shoulder is seen in 25% of recurrently unstable patients according to Hovelius *et al*. No difference in dominant and non-dominant extremities was noted.

9. c. **Diabetes mellitus**.
Adhesive capsulitis affects an estimated 2–5% of the population. Several medical conditions have been associated with idiopathic adhesive capsulitis including diabetes and hypothyroidism. The reported incidence in diabetics is between 10% and 36%. Patients with insulin-dependent diabetes tend to have more severe limitation of movement and are more resistant to non-surgical treatment than non-insulin diabetics.

10. e. **Medial scapular winging**.
The long thoracic nerve supplies serratus anterior, injury to which can result in medial translation of the scapular and the inferior angle rotated medially. Lateral scapular winging (lateral translation and the inferior angle rotated laterally) can occur as result of spinal accessory nerve palsy which supplies trapezius.

11. b. **Normal anatomic variant characterized by a cord-like MGHL and an absent anterosuperior labrum**.
A Buford complex is a normal anatomical variant seen in 1.5% of individuals. A Buford complex consists of a cord-like MGHL and absent anterosuperior labrum complex. It should not be 'repaired'. 'Repair' will result in decreased post-operative range of motion.

12. a. **Risk of dislocation**.
As part of a deltopectoral approach, the subscapularis is taken down off the humerus. This may be done trans-tendon, directly off bone, or with a lesser tuberosity osteotomy. In the initial post-operative period passive external rotation is limited to a maximum 30° to allow healing and protect the repair.

13. d. **Axillary**.
The most common nerve to be injured in a traumatic anterior shoulder dislocation is the axillary nerve. This is because of its close association with the glenohumeral joint and its course around the surgical neck of the humerus. Based on clinical and electromyography

(EMG) findings Visser *et al.* showed that the axillary nerve is injured in 42% of traumatic anterior dislocations.

14. **d. Extensor carpi radialis brevis.**
The patient has lateral epicondylitis (tennis elbow), which usually involves a microtear of extensor carpi radialis brevis (ECRB). Histologically the lesion that was consistently identified at surgery was immature fibroblastic and vascular infiltration (angiofibroblastic dysplasia) of the origin of ECRB.

15. **d. Anterior band of the medial ulnar collateral ligament.**
The anterior band provides the major contribution to valgus stability. The olecranon is an important stabilizer of the elbow in extension; at 25° flexion the olecranon is unlocked from its fossa and the ulnar collateral ligament becomes the most important stabilizer. The radial head is an important secondary stabilizer in flexion and extension. The posterior band of the medial ulnar collateral ligament is a secondary stabilizer at 30° of flexion. The transverse band plays no role in joint stability because it originates and inserts on the same bone.

16. **c. Late cocking.**
The late cocking and early acceleration phase of the overhead throw causes the greatest amount of valgus stress to the elbow. During this phase, the forearm lags behind the upper arm and generates valgus stress while the elbow is primarily dependent on the anterior band of the ulnar collateral ligament for stability. In deceleration, the elbow flexors are most active to prevent hyperextension.

17. **c. Activity modification.**
Distal clavicular osteolysis is an uncommon cause of shoulder pain that can occur after acute injury or repetitive microtrauma. Initial treatment is non-surgical and includes activity modification and ACJ steroid injection. Arthroscopic resection of the distal clavicle should be considered in patients refractory to non-operative treatment.

18. **a. Inferior glenohumeral.**
A humeral avulsion of the glenohumeral ligament (HAGL) lesion is a detachment of the inferior glenohumeral ligament (IGHL) off its humeral insertion. If missed, it can cause a failure of Bankart repair. The classic teaching is for repair via an open approach.

19. **d. External rotation deficit.**
Healing of the tuberosities and their attached rotator cuff tendons is crucial in functional outcome after arthroplasty. Failure to properly position tuberosity fragments in the horizontal plane may result in insurmountable post-operative motion restriction.

20. **a. Weakness in external rotation.**
Compression at the spinoglenoid notch will affect only the infraspinatus as the suprascapular nerve has already innervated the supraspinatus by this point. Compression at the suprascapular notch will affect both the supraspinatus and the infraspinatus. Prolonged impingement on the suprascapular nerve by a spinoglenoid cyst can result in atrophy of the infraspinatus muscles. This would show up as weakness in external rotation on examination. These cysts are associated with SLAP lesions and are formed

by a one-way valve effect, where synovial fluid can exit the joint into the cyst but not drain spontaneously.

21. b. Superior placement of the glenoid component.
Superior positioning of the glenoid component as well as superior tilt of the component with respect to the scapula can lead to scapular notching, with a resultant poorer outcome. Inferior tilt and proper placement of the glenoid component protects against notching.

22. e. Anteroinferior labral tear.
It has been shown in one study that 87% have an anterior glenoid labral tear (Bankart lesion), 79% had anterior capsular insufficiency, 68% had a Hill–Sachs lesion, 55% had glenohumeral ligament insufficiency, 14% had complete rotator cuff tears, 12% had posterior glenoid labral tears and 7% had SLAP tears.

23. c. Posterior interosseous nerve.
The posterior interosseous nerve is vulnerable as it winds around the neck of the radius within the supinator muscle. Fully supinating the forearm displaces the nerve laterally and posteriorly (away from the surgical site) at the same time more fully exposing the insertion of supinator.

24. b. Decreased shoulder muscle strength and endurance.
McKee found that patients who had non-operative treatment of displaced (> 2 cm) midshaft clavicle fractures had significant decrease in both strength and endurance of about 80% compared to the contralateral side. Range of motion (ROM) of the affected shoulder was unaffected.

25. e. Total elbow replacement.
The Larsen classification of the rheumatoid elbow is based on plain radiographs and is graded I–V:
   Grade I – soft tissue swelling and osteoporosis.
   Grade II – mild narrowing of the joint space and some marginal erosion.
   Grade III – significant joint space narrowing.
   Grade IV – integrity of subchondral plates is breached by deep erosions.
   Grade V – total joint destruction

26. b. Rotator cuff repair.
A shoulder dislocation in a patient >40 years commonly results in a rotator cuff tear. In a shoulder with an intact rotator cuff, the dye will remain in the glenohumeral joint. A rotator cuff tear allows the dye to leak into the subacromial space. The most appropriate treatment is a rotator cuff repair.

**27. e. Radial head arthroplasty, coronoid open reduction internal fixation,
        and lateral collateral ligament repair.**
A terrible triad of the elbow includes dislocation of the elbow with associated fractures of the radial head and the coronoid process. Ring *et al.* stressed that these injuries are prone to complications and advised against resection of the radial head due to instability,

and instead recommended a radial head replacement if too comminuted for open reduction and internal rotation (ORIF). Coronoid fractures compromise elbow stability as well and require open reduction and internal fixation as with the lateral collateral ligament.

28. a.   **Ligament avulsion off the humeral origin.**
The LUCL is most commonly injured at the proximal origin. McKee *et al.* noted that in 62 consecutive operative elbow dislocations and fracture/dislocations, the LUCL was ruptured in all of the patients, proximally in 32, bony avulsion proximally in 5, midsubstance rupture in 18, ulnar detachment in 3, ulnar bony avulsion in 1 and combined patterns in 3.

29. a.   **Suprascapular-axillary.**
Surgical fixation of a scapular neck fracture is performed via a posterior approach to the scapular/glenoid. The internervous plane is between the infraspinatus (suprascapular nerve) and the teres minor (axillary nerve). The posterior branch of the axillary nerve has intimate association with the inferior aspects of the glenoid and shoulder joint capsule, and can be found in the interval between teres minor and teres major, which may place it at particular risk during a posterior approach to the shoulder.

30. c.   **Internal rotation (IR) 30°, Flexion 30°, Abduction 30°.**
Shoulder arthrodesis should be performed so that the arm rests comfortably at the side without scapular winging and so that the hand can be brought easily to the mouth and perineum.

EMQs

1. 1. **b. Spinal accessory nerve.** 2. **c. Long thoracic nerve.** 3. **g. Radial nerve.**
Injury to the spinal accessory nerve which supplies trapezius can result in shoulder depression with scapular lateral translation and the inferior angle rotating laterally because of the unopposed action of serratus anterior.

There are four supraclavicular branches of the brachial plexus: long thoracic nerve, dorsal scapular nerve, suprascapular nerve, nerve to subclavius.

In elbow arthroscopy the radial nerve is only 4 mm from the anterolateral portal, while the median nerve is 11 mm away from the anteromedial portal. The ulnar nerve is only at risk on the medial side of the elbow.

2. 1. **c. Middle glenohumeral ligament (MGHL).** 2. **d. Anterior band of the inferior glenohumeral ligament (IGHL).** 3. **h. Subscapularis.**
There are static and dynamic stabilizers of the shoulder. Static restraints: articular anatomy, glenoid labrum, capsule, ligaments, negative pressure. Dynamic restraints: rotator cuff, biceps. The MGHL (absent in up to 40%) is a primary restraint to anterior translation of the externally rotated arm in the midrange of abduction.

The anterior band of the IGHL is the primary restraint to anterior/inferior translation of the head with the shoulder abducted to 90° and in maximum external rotation (ER).

The posterior band of the IGHL is the most important restraint to posterior subluxation of the GHL with the shoulder in 90° of flexion and internal rotation (IR). In ER, the subscapularis is an important dynamic stabilizer to posterior subluxation.

The superior glenohumeral ligament functions as a primary restraint to ER in the adducted arm.

3. 1. **f. Serendipity view.** 2. **a. Supraspinatus outlet view.** 3. **g. Stryker notch view.**
The different radiographic views are taken for – acromion morphology (supraspinatus outlet view), Hill–Sachs lesion (anteroposterior (AP) in internal rotation (IR), Stryker notch view), acromioclavicular joint (ACJ) (Zanca), sternoclavicular joint (SCJ) (serendipity), bony bankart (Garth), glenohumeral joint space (true anteroposterior (AP)), anterior/posterior dislocation (axillary view).

4. 1. **a. Lateral epicondylitis.** 2. **f. Posterior interosseous syndrome.** 3. **d. Posterolateral rotatory instability.**
Posterior interosseous nerve (PIN) compression causes lateral elbow pain and ulnar drift with wrist extension as extensor carpi radialis longus (ECRL) is innervated proximal to PIN branch. Radial tunnel syndrome is a pain only problem without motor or sensory dysfunction.

Iatrogenic injury to the lateral ulnar collateral ligament, the main ligament implicated in posterolateral rotatory instability (PLRI) is a complication of a lateral release for tennis elbow. The anterior band of the medial collateral ligament is implicated in valgus instability.

5. 1. **a. Lateral collateral ligament.** 2. **b. Lateral ulnar collateral ligament.** 3. **h. Ulnar collateral ligament.**
Posterolateral rotatory instability (PLRI) of the elbow describes a rotational displacement as the ulna supinates past its normal limit and the radiocapitellar joint subluxes

posterolaterally, permitting the coronoid process to slide beneath the trochlea. The lateral ulnar collateral ligament has been shown to be the essential lesion responsible for PLRI. The medial collateral ligament (of which the anterior bundle (ulnar collateral) is the most important) is the primary restraint to valgus instability. The posterolateral capsule and radial collateral ligament may be disrupted in a complete posterolateral dislocation but are not essential injuries for PLRI.

6. 1. **i. Adhesive capsulitis**. 2. **g. Subcoracoid impingement**. 3. **d. Thoracic outlet syndrome**.

Adhesive capsulitis is characterized by pain (particularly at night) and decreased active and passive range of motion (especially external rotation (ER)). Subcoracoid impingement (subscapularis impingement between the coracoid and lesser tuberosity) presents with anterior shoulder pain, the position of maximal discomfort 120–130° of forward flexion and internal rotation. On a CT scan a coracohumeral distance of <6 mm is considered abnormal. A local anaesthetic injection to the subcoracoid space should eliminate symptoms.

Thoracic outlet syndrome is associated with clavicle malunion (also scalene muscle abnormality, cervical rib). It most often affects subclavian artery, vein and the lower trunk (C8 and T1) of the brachial plexus. Abduction and ER with the neck rotated away leads to loss of pulse and reproduction of symptoms (Wright test).

7. 1. **c. Subscapularis repair**. 2. **i. Reverse type total shoulder arthroplasty**. 3. **g. Latissimus dorsi tendon transfer**.

After a total shoulder arthroplasty external rotation, as well as active internal rotation, is limited to protect the subscapularis repair. This patient recruited his subscapularis rising from the chair. Initial treatment should be surgical repair.

A reverse type prosthesis is indicated for the second patient. The main complication associated with an unconstrained total shoulder arthroplasty in the presence of a cuff-tear arthropathy is loosening of the glenoid component.

The third patient is a candidate for a latissimus dorsi tendon transfer. The best outcome is achieved when the subscapularis is intact and there is full passive range of motion (ROM).

8. 1. **f. Posterior approach to the shoulder**. 2. **f. Posterior approach to the shoulder**. 3. **g. Lateral approach to the shoulder**.

The posterior approach to the shoulder is the interval between infraspinatus (suprascapular nerve) and teres minor (axillary nerve). It is the approach of choice for posterior glenoid, scapular fracture fixation. The lateral approach to the shoulder is a deltoid split through the anterior raphe. It is used for fixation of greater tuberosity fractures.

9. 1. **j. Belly press**. 2. **h. Hornblower's sign**. 3. **c. Hawkin's sign**.

The subscapularis has two portions, the upper portion innervated by the upper subscapular nerve (C5) and the lower portion from the lower subscapular nerve (C5–C6). The lift-off test is more accurate for the lower portion of the subscapularis and the belly press test more sensitive for the upper portion.

Hornblower's sign (shoulder to 90° abduction, 90° external rotation and ask patient to hold position); if the arm falls into internal rotation it suggests a tear of teres minor.

10. 1. **c. Pectoralis major rupture**. 2. **i. Glenohumeral osteoarthritis**. 3. **h. Subscapularis rupture**.

Mechanism of injury is excessive tension on a maximally eccentrically contracted muscle. Bruising on the upper arm (rather than chest wall) suggests detachment at the humeral insertion rather than an intrasubstance tear.

Loss of external rotation can lead to degenerative joint disease following an anterior stabilization procedure. In time, this patient's shoulder may show increased posterior glenohumeral wear.

Subscapularis tendon tears are a complication of open anterior stabilization surgery where subscapularis has been detached as part of the approach. The patient will have anterior shoulder pain and may report a sensation of instability. The lift-off test usually is positive.

11. 1. **b. SLAP type II**. 2. **d. SLAP type IV**. 3. **i. Biceps tendon subluxation**.

Snyder originally described four types of SLAP lesion. Type 1 biceps fraying, type II detachment of the biceps anchor, type III bucket handle tear, superior labral tear, intact biceps, in type IV it extends into the biceps tendon. The classification has since been expanded to include SLAP lesions associated with shoulder instability. Type II is the most common clinically significant type.

Biceps tendon subluxation is commonly associated with a subscapularis tear. A tear of the coracohumeral ligament or transverse humeral ligament may also result in subluxation.

12. 1. **d. Open reduction and internal fixation (ORIF)**. 2. **d. Open reductor and internal fixator (ORIF)**. 3. **d. Open reduction and internal fixation (ORIF)**.

Displacement of the greater tuberosity >5 mm can result in symptoms of pain and limitation of movement. Osteonecrosis or loss of fixation is particularly likely after a head-split fracture. However, in a young patient, ORIF should be attempted. A good result with ORIF is seen in valgus impacted fractures with low rates of avascular necrosis (AVN) if the posteromedial component is intact thus preserving the intraosseous blood supply.

13. 1. **b. Triangular interval**. 2. **b. Triangular interval**. 3. **a. Triangular space**.

The quadrangular space is bordered by teres minor (superiorly), teres major (inferiorly), long head triceps (medially), and the humeral shaft (laterally). It contains the axillary nerve and posterior circumflex humeral vessels. The triangular space is bordered by teres minor (superiorly), teres major (inferiorly), and long head triceps (laterally). It contains the circumflex scapular vessels. The triangular interval is bordered by teres major (superiorly), long head triceps (medially) and humerus (laterally). It contains the profunda brachii artery and radial nerve.

14. 1. **d. Open reduction and internal fixation (ORIF)**. 2. **e. Radial head replacement**. 3. **j. Medial ligament reconstruction**.

The examination and radiograph suggest that displacement of the fragment is great enough (>2 mm) to create a mechanical block. The prefered treatment is ORIF.

The second patient has an Essex-Lopresti fracture. Excision of the radial head without replacement will result in the radius migrating proximally causing wrist pain and loss of motion.

Repetitive valgus stress can result in rupture of the anterior band of the medial collateral ligament. Patients may complain of ulnar nerve symptoms. If initial non-operative management fails, especially in high level athletes, then medial collateral ligament reconstruction is favoured over direct repair.

15. 1. **e. Lateral condyle**. 2. **a. Capitellum**. 3. **g. Trochlea**.
Cubitis valgus deformity following a lateral condyle fracture can lead to tardy ulnar nerve palsy.

Osteochondritis dissecans is localized fragmentation of the bone and overlying cartilage of the capitellum; it frequently progresses to loose body formation, and sometimes progresses to post-traumatic arthritis. It tends to occur in patients 10–16 years of age.

'CRITOL' can be used to remember the chronological sequence of elbow ossification: capitellum – 2 years; radial head – 4 years; internal epicondyle – 6 years; trochlea – 8 years; olecranon – 10 years; lateral epicondyle –12 years.

Selected references

Frankle MA, Greenwald DP, Markee BA, Ondrovic LE, Lee WE 3rd. Biomechanical effects of malposition of tuberosity fragments on the humeral prosthetic reconstruction for four-part proximal humerus fractures. *J Shoulder Elbow Surg* 2001; **10**(4): 321–6.

Hoppenfeld S, deBoer P, Buckley R. *Surgical Exposures in Orthopaedics: The Anatomic Approach*, 3rd edn. Philadelphia, Lippincott Williams and Wilkins, 2009.

Hovelius L, Olofsson A, Sandström B, *et al*. Nonoperative treatment of primary anterior shoulder dislocation in patients forty years of age and younger. A prospective twenty-five-year follow-up. *J Bone Joint Surg Am* 2008; **90**(5): 945–52.

McKee MD, Pedersen EM, Jones C *et al*. Deficits following non-operative treatment of displaced midshaft clavicular fractures. *J Bone Joint Surg Am* 2006; **88**(1): 35–40.

McKee MD, Pugh DM, Wild LM *et al*. Standard surgical protocol to treat elbow dislocations with radial head and coronoid fractures: surgical technique. *J Bone Joint Surg Am* 2005; **87**: 22–32.

McKee MD, Schemitsch EH, Sala MJ, O'driscoll SW. The pathoanatomy of lateral ligamentous disruption in complex elbow instability. *J Shoulder Elbow Surg* 2003; **12**: 391–6.

Miller BS, Joseph TA, Noonan TJ, Horan MP, Hawkins RJ. Rupture of the subscapularis tendon after shoulder arthroplasty: diagnosis, treatment, and outcome. *J Shoulder Elbow Surg* 2005; **14**(5): 492–6.

Miller MJ. *Review of Orthopaedics*, 5th edn. Philadelphia, Elsevier, 2008.

Millett PJ, Clavert P, Hatch GF 3rd, Warner JJ. Recurrent posterior shoulder instability. *J Am Acad Orthop Surg* 2006; **14**: 464–76.

Nirschl RP, Pettrone FA. Tennis elbow: the surgical treatment of lateral epicondylitis. *J Bone Joint Surg Am* 1979; **61**: 832–9.

Ring D, Jupiter JB, Zilberfarb J. Posterior dislocation of the elbow with fractures of the radial head and coronoid. *J Bone Joint Surg Am* 2002; **84**: 547–51.

Visser CP, Coene LN, Brand R, Tavy DL. The incidence of nerve injury in anterior dislocation of the shoulder and its influence on functional recovery. A prospective clinical and EMG study. *J Bone Joint Surg Br* 1999; **81**(4): 679–85.

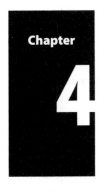

Spine: Questions

Zaher Dannawi and Rajiv A. Bajekal

MCQs

1. **All of the following statements regarding thoracolumbar trauma are true except?**
   a. Instability of a vertebral fracture can be determined by loss of vertebral height >50%.
   b. There is no direct relationship between canal compromise and neurological deficit.
   c. Instability of injuries can be determined by further neurological deterioration under normal physiological load.
   d. Widening of the interpedicular distance on plain radiograph can indicate a burst fracture.
   e. In a thoracic burst fracture, a thoracolumbar orthosis is indicated if there is <50% loss of vertebral body height and >30% kyphosis.

2. **All of the following statements regarding curve progression in adolescent idiopathic scoliosis are true except?**
   a. With curves of 20–29°, 40% of patients who are Risser 0–1 are at risk of curve progression.
   b. With curves of 20–29°, 22% of patients who are Risser 2–4 progress.
   c. After skeletal maturity, a lumbar curve >35° can progress by 1–2°/year.
   d. A late curve progression in males is more common than in females.
   e. A rapid curve progression in females occurs before menarche and before Risser 1.

3. **During an anterior instrumented fusion of the lumbar spine through a left-sided retroperitoneal approach, all of the following statements are correct except?**
   a. The ureter is adherent to the posterior peritoneum and falls away from the psoas through the dissection.
   b. The sympathetic trunk, lying longitudinally along the lateral border of the psoas, is at risk during this procedure.
   c. The ilioinguinal nerve emerges from the lateral border of the psoas and travels to the quadratus lumborium.
   d. A cold and pale right foot is a recognized post-operative examination finding.
   e. The genitofemoral nerve lies on the anteromedial surface of the psoas.

4. **All of the following statements regarding scoliosis in neurofibromatosis (NF) are true except?**
   a. Non-dystrophic deformities are indistinguishable from idiopathic scoliosis.

Postgraduate Orthopaedics, ed. Kesavan Sri-Ram. Published by Cambridge University Press.
© Cambridge University Press 2012.

b. The typical curve of NF-1 is characterized by a short and sharp curvature.

c. Scalloping of the vertebral bodies with enlargement of the neural foramina are features of a dystrophic curve.

d. Marked rotation of the apical vertebra with pencilling of the ribs can often be found in dystrophic curves.

e. Neurological deficit associated with compression from neurofibromata or kyphoscoliosis is uncommon.

5. **Which of the following is true regarding superior mesenteric artery (SMA) syndrome?**
   a. The condition often occurs in overweight female patients.
   b. This syndrome is also known as cast syndrome.
   c. This condition occurs following curve correction as a result of an increase in the angle between the aorta and the superior mesenteric artery.
   d. The condition is due to an ischaemic event of the SMA.
   e. This is a surgical emergency requiring an early laparotomy +/− duodenojejunostomy.

6. **A 46-year-old man presents to the clinic with severe back pain. All of the following are consistent with non-organic signs except?**
   a. Discrepancy between findings on supine and sitting straight leg raising tests.
   b. Disproportionate facial expressions or tremor during examination.
   c. Low back pain on passive rotation of shoulders and pelvis in the same plane.
   d. According to Waddell et al, non-organic signs should be equated with malingering or the presence of a psychological problem.
   e. Non-dermatomal sensory loss.

7. **A 32-year-old man presents with a 2 month history of back and right-sided leg pain. He walked with a right Trendelenburg gait. The most likely diagnosis is?**
   a. An ipsilateral paracentral disc herniation at L3–L4.
   b. An ipsilateral paracentral disc herniation at L5–S1.
   c. An ipsilateral far lateral disc herniation at L4–L5.
   d. An ipsilateral far lateral disc herniation at L5–S1.
   e. An ipsilateral foraminal disc herniation at L4–L5.

8. **Which of the following is incorrect regarding spinal tuberculosis?**
   a. It originates underneath the anterior longitudinal ligament and can cause destruction of several contiguous levels.
   b. It can cause skip lesions at non-contiguous segments in 15% of the cases.
   c. In the early disease process, the disc spaces are relatively preserved.
   d. Kyphosis and Pott paraplegia are late sequelae.
   e. Spinal cord injury occurring secondary to a bony sequestra carries a good prognosis.

9. **A 58-year-old lady with rheumatoid arthritis (RA) presents with neck pain and occipital headache. Which of the following is true regarding her condition?**
   a. Atlantoaxial subluxation occurs in 25% of cases of RA as the result of pannus formation.
   b. An anterior atlantodens interval (ADI) of more than 3.5 mm on flexion-extension views indicates instability and an absolute indication for surgery.

   c. A space available for the cord (SAC) of less than 14 mm or an ADI of more than 9–10 mm is an indication for spinal stabilization.

   d. A Ranawat (C1–C2) index of <17 mm is consistent with basilar invagination.

   e. A subaxial subluxation of >4 mm is not indicative of cord compression.

10. A 26-year-old builder underwent an L4–L5 discectomy 12 months ago. He continues to experience pain in his right leg. Systemically he is well in himself. Gadolinium-enhanced MRI scans showed enhancement adjacent to the right L5 root. There is no fluid collection. What is the most likely diagnosis?
   a. L4–L5 discitis.
   b. Recurrent right L4–L5 disc herniation.
   c. Epidural abscess.
   d. Right L5 perineural fibrosis.
   e. Schwannoma of the right L5 root.

11. A 19-year-old patient presents with low back pain. Which of the following is a 'yellow flag' rather than a 'red flag'?
   a. Age of the patient.
   b. Poor appetite.
   c. History of intravenous drug use.
   d. Failure to improve with rest, supine position or therapy.
   e. Pain avoidance.

12. A 12-year-old girl with scoliosis was found to have a fluid-filled cavity within the spinal cord on a routine preoperative MRI scan. All of the following are true regarding the spinal cord finding except?
   a. Craniocervical junction abnormalities are predisposing factors.
   b. Scoliosis is reported in 25–85% of syringomyelia cases.
   c. Scoliosis with syringomyelia has been characterized by 44–50% incidence of left thoracic curves.
   d. Proprioception and vibration sensation are usually not affected.
   e. Decompression of the syrinx in patients above the age of 10 years will improve or stabilize the scoliotic curve.

13. A 33-year-old male is involved in a road traffic accident sustaining a fracture dislocation of the cervical spine. He has absent motor function, absent sensation and anal tone. The bulbocavernous reflex is intact. Which of the following best describes this spinal cord injury pattern?
   a. Central cord syndrome.
   b. Incomplete spinal cord injury.
   c. Complete spinal cord injury.
   d. Neurogenic shock.
   e. Spinal shock.

14. A 20-year-old cyclist was hit by a car sustaining a spinal cord injury. He has an MRC 5 in his deltoids and biceps, MRC 0 in his wrist extensors, flexors and triceps. He has

an absent anal tone and perianal sensation. He has absent tone and power in his lower limbs. How would you define this patient's neurological injury?
a. Incomplete C5.
b. Complete C5.
c. Complete C6.
d. Incomplete C6.
e. Incomplete C7.

15. All of the following can be present with diastematomyelia except?
    a. Tethering of the cord.
    b. Intrapedicular widening.
    c. Enlarged intervertebral foramina.
    d. Neurological deficit.
    e. Diplomyelia.

16. An MRI of a 32-year-old patient shows a left foraminal disc herniation of the L5–S1 disc. Which of the following is unlikely to be present?
    a. Left lateral foot numbness.
    b. Left extensor hallucis longus (EHL) weakness.
    c. Left dorsomedial foot numbness.
    d. Left lateral calf numbness.
    e. Left extensor digitorum longus (EDL) weakness.

17. All of the following are true of scoliosis except?
    a. Idiopathic adolescent curves are commonly right thoracic.
    b. A thoracic curve >50° will progress by 1–2°/year after skeletal maturity.
    c. Infantile scoliosis commonly affects girls and is usually left-sided.
    d. Infantile scoliosis is associated with plagiocephaly.
    e. A rib vertebral angle (RVA) of >20° is associated with a high rate of progression.

18. In central canal stenosis of the lumbar spine, all of the following are true except?
    a. It is more common in men.
    b. Acquired stenosis is the more common type.
    c. Tension signs are usually positive.
    d. A history of radiating leg pain in a dermatomal distribution is relatively uncommon.
    e. Can occur as a result of Paget's disease.

19. A 19-year-old medical student presents with a Scheuermann's kyphosis in the thoracic spine with a Cobb angle of 85° between T5 and T12. All of the following are correct except?
    a. The condition is often accompanied by a lumbar hyperlordosis.
    b. This is the most common cause of thoracic back pain in adolescents.
    c. An MRI scan should be part of a routine preoperative workup.
    d. A posterior instrumentation should stop at the distal most tilted vertebra.
    e. At surgery, flavectomy (ligamentum flavum excision) should be performed at the apex of the curve.

20. **All of the following are true regarding intervertebral disc disease except?**
    a. With age, the proteoglycan (PG) synthesis decreases; however, the PG concentration increases due to the drop in the water content.
    b. With age, there is no change in the absolute quantity of collagen.
    c. Disc stimulation studies (discogram) have shown that when stimulated, normal discs do not cause pain.
    d. With age there is a decrease in type I and an increase in type III collagen in the annulus.
    e. Reproduction of pain does not correlate with disc degeneration but with the degree of disc fissuring.

21. **All of the following are true for hangman's fracture except?**
    a. It is a traumatic spondylolisthesis of C2 on C3 as a result of bilateral fracture of C2 pars or pedicles.
    b. The mechanism of injury is a primary hyperflexion of the neck.
    c. Type IIA fracture has a significant angulation without displacement.
    d. Type I fracture has an intact C2/C3 disc.
    e. A C2/C3 fusion is indicated for a type III fracture.

22. **A 29-year-old restrained front seat passenger was involved in a road traffic accident, sustaining a flexion-distraction injury of L1. Which of the following is true regarding this fracture?**
    a. Gastrointestinal injuries occur in 25% of cases.
    b. A bony chance fracture has a high non-union rate compared to the ligamentous injury.
    c. A ligamentous chance fracture should be treated using a distraction construct with three levels above and two levels below the fracture.
    d. A ligamentous chance fracture should be treated using a compression construct with one level above and one level below the fracture.
    e. It is commonly associated with neurological deficit.

23. **All of the following are true of Klippel–Feil syndrome except?**
    a. It is a congenital failure of segmentation of the cervical spine.
    b. It is associated with Sprengel's shoulder and other congenital abnormalities.
    c. The classic triad of low posterior hairline, short neck and reduced range of movement is seen in less than 50% of the cases.
    d. Flexion/extension of the C-spine is often reduced.
    e. Scoliosis is present in 60% of cases.

24. **What constitutes a spinal motion segment?**
    a. A disc and the facet joints at that level.
    b. A disc and the vertebrae above and below, including their interlocking facet joints.
    c. A section of the spine involved in a physiological curve with the similar function (i.e. thoracic kyphosis).
    d. A vertebral body and the disc above.
    e. A disc and the vertebrae above and below, including their interlocking facet joints and surrounding musculature.

25. A 23-year-old motorcyclist was involved in a road traffic accident. He was brought to the A&E unconscious with multiple injuries. It is anticipated that he will remain unconscious and unassessable for more than 48 hours. Which cervical radiological spinal clearance imaging should be undertaken?
    a. Anteroposterior (AP) and lateral radiographs of the C-spine.
    b. Helical CT scan with a 5–6 mm slice from the base of the skull to at least T1.
    c. MRI scans of the neck.
    d. Helical CT scan with a 2–3 mm slice from the base of the skull to at least T1.
    e. Lateral radiograph of the C-spine +/− swimmer's view if the former is inadequate.

26. A 10-year-old-girl presents with a painful scoliosis. Radiographs showed a 35° right thoracic scoliosis with a radiolucent nidus <1 cm at the apex of the curve. Which of the following is incorrect regarding this spinal lesion?
    a. Pain is usually due to prostaglandin found in the nidus.
    b. CT scan is the investigation of choice to identify the nidus.
    c. Bone scan is always hot with intense uptake.
    d. Medical management with non-steroidal anti-inflammatory drugs (NSAIDs) is a satisfactory treatment modality in this case.
    e. The natural history of this condition is that of spontaneous resolution.

27. A 50-year-old man presents with difficulty mobilizing and clumsiness buttoning his shirt. He had a fixed cervical kyphosis of 15°. An MRI scan showed a central disc herniation at C5–C6 with signal changes within the cord. What is the next appropriate management step?
    a. Observation.
    b. Posterior decompression.
    c. Posterior decompression and fusion.
    d. Anterior cervical decompression and fusion.
    e. Posterior osteotomy to correct the kyphosis followed by posterior fusion.

28. Which of the following is incorrect regarding the anterolateral approach (Smith–Robinson) to the cervical spine?
    a. The platysma and external jugular vein are the only structures superficial to the superficial fascia.
    b. The superior and inferior thyroid vessels run from the carotid sheath through the pretracheal fascia to the midline.
    c. The sympathetic chain lies on the longus colli muscle lateral to the vertebral body.
    d. Recurrent laryngeal nerve injury risk is lower at the lower C-spine levels (C6–C7).
    e. Dysphagia occurs more commonly at the upper C-spine levels (C3–C4).

29. All of the following are true regarding atlantoaxial rotatory instability except:
    a. It is a common cause of childhood torticollis.
    b. It is associated with Down syndrome.
    c. It can occur secondary to Grisel's syndrome.
    d. A type II rotator subluxation indicates an insufficiency of the transverse and alar ligaments.
    e. In a type III rotatory subluxation, both joints are anteriorly subluxed with an atlantodens interval of >5 mm.

30. **The central cord syndrome is due to?**
    a. A fall on a flexed neck.
    b. Hyperextension injury on a background of a herniated disc.
    c. A hyperextension injury in a patient with a facet joint hypertrophy and thickened ligamentum flavum.
    d. An anterior spinal artery lesion.
    e. Vitamin B12 deficiency.

EMQs

1. **Spinal cord injuries**
   a. Central cord syndrome
   b. Anterior cord syndrome
   c. Brown-Séquard syndrome
   d. Posterior cord syndrome
   e. Cauda equina syndrome
   f. Root injury
   g. Complete cord injury

Which of the options above is best described in each of the following statements? Each option may be used once, more than once or not at all.
   1. A 78-year-old man fell down the stairs sustaining an injury to the neck. He has an MRC grade 3 in his upper limbs and MRC grade 4 in his lower limbs.
   2. A 36-year-old man was stabbed in the right posterior thorax. He has loss of motor function and proprioception on the right side with intact motor power with some sensory loss on the left side.
   3. A 14-year-old girl with adolescent idiopathic scoliosis was unable to move her legs following an anterior approach to the thoracolumbar spine. Proprioception and vibration sense were preserved.

2. **Findings in lumbar disc disease**
   a. Right paracentral L3/L4 disc herniation
   b. Right foraminal L3/L4 disc herniation
   c. Right paracentral L4/L5 disc herniation
   d. Right far lateral L4/L5 disc herniation
   e. Right foraminal L5/S1 disc herniation
   f. Right posterolateral L5/S1 disc herniation

Which of the options above is best described in each of the following statements? Each option may be used once, more than once or not at all.
   1. A 32-year-old man presents with sensory loss over the right medial calf with an MRC grade 3 in the right tibialis anterior. He was operated through a Wiltse approach.
   2. A 23-year-old lady presents with sensory loss over the lateral aspect of her right leg and dorsal foot with an MRC grade 4 in the right extensor hallucis longus. She was told that this is the most common location of a disc herniation.
   3. A 25-year-old builder presents with numbness over the lateral aspect of his right foot. With an MRC grade 3 in his right gastro-soleus complex.

3. **Spondylolisthesis**
   a. Dysplastic
   b. Isthmic type IIA
   c. Isthmic type IIB
   d. Degenerative at L4/L5
   e. Traumatic
   f. Pathological

g. Postsurgical
h. Degenerative at L5/S1

Which of the options above is best described in each of the following statements? Each option may be used once, more than once or not at all.

1. An 11-year-old girl presents with back pain. She was found to have a grade I anterolisthesis of L5 on S1 with malorientated facets.
2. A 48-year-old diabetic lady presents with back pain and reduced sensation in the L5 dermatome with an MRC grade 3 in the extensor hallucis longus (EHL).
3. A 20-year-old ballet dancer presents with back pain. She was found to have an elongated pars.

4. **Spinal cord injury**
   a. C4
   b. C5
   c. C6
   d. C7
   e. C8
   f. T1
   g. T2–T12

Which of the functional levels above is best described in each of the following statements? Each option may be used once, more than once or not at all.

1. A 20-year-old male sustained a fracture dislocation of the cervical spine. He can eat and dress up but is unable to actively straighten his arm.
2. Patients at this level can cut meat but are unable to grasp.
3. Patients at this level can transfer independently. Manual wheelchairs and the use of flexor hinge wrist-hand orthosis can be operated at this level.

5. **Primary tumours**
   a. Osteoid osteoma
   b. Osteoblastoma
   c. Aneurysmal bone cyst
   d. Haemangioma
   e. Eosinophilic granuloma
   f. Giant cell tumour
   g. Plasmacytoma

Which of the options above is best described in each of the following statements? Each option may be used once, more than once or not at all.

1. An 8-year-old boy presents with mid-thoracic back pain. Radiographs of his spine showed a vertebra plana at T10.
2. A 40-year-old man sustained a wedge fracture of L1 following a fall. Jailhouse striations of the vertebra were also seen.
3. A high recurrence rate is reported following surgical excision of this tumour.

6. **Treatment of spinal tumours**
   a. Observation
   b. Radiotherapy

   c. Chemotherapy +/− local radiation
   d. Curettage
   e. Palliative care
   f. Wide-margin surgical resection +/− radiotherapy
   g. CT-guided radiofrequency ablation therapy
   h. Neoadjuvant chemotherapy/surgery/chemotherapy

Which of the options above is best described in each of the following statements? Each option may be used once, more than once or not at all.

   1. A 14-year-old boy has had back pain for the last 8 months that has failed to improve with observation and non-steroidal anti-inflammatory medications. Radiographs showed a reactive bone around a 1 cm radiolucent nidus in the lamina of L1.
   2. A 54-year-old-male presented with a 3 month history of back pain. Radiographs showed ivory vertebrae. Histology showed a mixed small round cell infiltrate.
   3. A 45-year-old lady presented with abdominal pain. A mass was palpable on rectal exam. Radiographs showed a lytic lesion of the anterior sacrum. Histology revealed cells with a foamy physaliferous appearance.

7. Back pain
   a. Mechanical back pain
   b. Cauda equina syndrome
   c. Spondylolisthesis
   d. Degenerative lumbar disc disease
   e. Normal discs
   f. Vascular claudication
   g. Spinal stenosis
   h. Unrecognized fracture
   i. Ankylosing spondylitis

Which of the options above is best described in each of the following statements? Each option may be used once, more than once or not at all.

   1. A 32-year-old man presents with low back pain, lower extremity numbness and urinary retention. He is able to walk but is in pain. A straight leg raise results in increased back pain, and examination reveals that perianal sensation is decreased. Placement of a urinary catheter results in 500 ml of urine.
   2. A 74-year-old man presents with bilateral calf pain in a distal–proximal direction. He gets symptom relief on lying flat.
   3. A 68-year-old man presents with buttock and bilateral leg pain made worse by walking and relieved on bending forward.

8. Cervical fracture/dislocation
   a. Jefferson's fracture
   b. Odontoid fracture
   c. Hangman's fracture
   d. Wedge compression fracture
   e. Clay shoveller's fracture
   f. Flexion "teardrop" fracture

g. Unilateral facet dislocation
h. Bilateral facet dislocation
i. Whiplash injury

Which of the options above is best described in each of the following statements? Each option may be used once, more than once or not at all.
1. A 40-year-old man dived into a shallow pool sustaining a fracture at C5. He was found to be quadriplegic with loss of anterior column sensation.
2. This injury is due to axial load and has a low incidence of neurological injury.
3. A 55-year-old woman has significant neck pain after falling and striking her head. Radiographs of her C-spine demonstrated the "bow tie sign".

9. Scoliosis treatment
a. Boston brace
b. Milwaukee brace
c. Posterior instrumented fusion of the thoracic curve
d. Anterior or posterior fusion of the lumbar curve
e. Anterior release followed by posterior instrumentation of the thoracic curve
f. Growth rods application
g. Spinal fusion down to pelvis
h. Posterior instrumented fusion of the thoracic and lumbar curve
i. Hemivertebrectomy

Which of the options above is best described in each of the following statements? Each option may be used once, more than once or not at all.
1. A 15-year-old girl presents with a right thoracic curve of 55° and a lumbar curve of 40°. On the bending views, the thoracic curve corrects to 33° and the lumbar to 18° with no significant apical vertebral rotation.
2. A 12-year-old presents with a right low thoracic curve (apex at T10) of 35°. She is still premenarchal.
3. A 15-year-old wheelchair user boy with cerebral palsy presents with a 70° lumbar curve with increase pelvic obliquity.

10. Pathology in the spine
a. Rheumatoid spondylitis
b. Ankylosing spondylitis
c. Diffuse idiopathic skeletal hyperostosis (DISH)
d. Ossification of the posterior longitudinal ligament (OPLL)
e. Peripheral neuropathy
f. Osteoporosis
g. Destructive spondyloarthropathy

Which of the options above is best described in each of the following statements? Each option may be used once, more than once or not at all.
1. A 70-year-old diabetic male presents with back pain and stiffness. Plain radiographs of the thoracolumbar spine showed the presence of non-marginal osteophytes at three successive levels.

2. A 48-year-old haemodialysis patient presents with back pain. Radiographs of the thoracolumbar spine showed a destruction of three adjacent vertebrae and two intervening discs.
3. A 38-year-old male presents with an insidious onset of back pain. Spine radiographs revealed the presence of vertical osteophytes.

11. **Neurological levels**
    a. T10
    b. T11
    c. T12
    d. L1
    e. L2
    f. L3
    g. L4
    h. L5
    i. S1
    j. S2

Which of the options above is best described in each of the following statements? Each option may be used once, more than once or not at all.
1. A 22-year-old presents with numbness over his left medial malleolus.
2. A 48-year-old presents with weakness in his extensor hallucis longus.
3. A 38-year-old is found to have an absent ankle jerk reflex.

12. **Radiological parameters**
    a. McRae
    b. Ranawat
    c. Space available for the cord (SAC)
    d. Chamberlain
    e. Atlantodens interval (ADI)
    f. McGregor
    g. Pavlov
    h. Wackenheim

Which of the options above is best described in each of the following statements? Each option may be used once, more than once or not at all.
1. A value less than 0.80 is considered a risk factor for neurological injury after minor trauma.
2. A value less than 14 mm is considered a risk factor for neurological injury in patients with rheumatoid arthritis.
3. This is a line drawn from the centre of the C2 pedicle to the C1 arch.

13. **Spinal tracts**
    a. Dorsal column
    b. Lateral spinothalamic tract
    c. Anterior spinothalamic tract
    d. Lateral corticospinal tract

    e. Ventral corticospinal tract
    f. Dorsal spinocerebellar tract
    g. Ventral spinocerebellar tract

Which of the options above is best described in each of the following statements? Each option may be used once, more than once or not at all.
1. This tract conveys temperature sensation.
2. This tract conveys proprioceptive information of the lower limbs from muscle spindles.
3. This tract is also known as the crossed pyramidal tract.

14. **Special examination tests**
    a. Babinski reflex
    b. Spurling's test
    c. Hoffman's test
    d. Inverted radial reflex
    e. Lhermitte's sign
    f. Oppenheim test
    g. Adam's test
    h. Schober's test
    i. FABER test
    j. Femoral stretch test
    k. Lasegue test
    l. Bowstring test

Which of the options above is best described in each of the following statements? Each option may be used once, more than once or not at all.
1. This involves applying pressure in the popliteal fossa.
2. This involves flexion of the cervical spine.
3. This involves quickly snapping or flicking the middle fingernail.

15. **Percentages relating to the spine**
    a. 0%
    b. 0–1%
    c. 1–2%
    d. 5%
    e. 10%
    f. 20%
    g. 30%
    h. 40%
    i. 50%
1. The approximate incidence of lumbar herniated nucleus pulposus in asymptomatic patients less than 60 years of age.
2. The risk of neurological deficit after idiopathic scoliosis surgery.
3. The risk of concomitant cervical injury after a hangman's fracture (traumatic spondylolithesis of the axis).

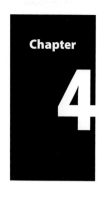

Spine: Answers

Zaher Dannawi and Rajiv A. Bajekal

MCQs

1. **e. In a thoracic burst fracture, a thoracolumbar orthosis is indicated if there is <50% loss of vertebral body height and >30% kyphosis.**
A thoracolumbar orthosis can be indicated in patients who are neurologically intact with a kyphosis <30%, a loss of vertebral body height <50% and with intact posterior elements. There is no direct relationship between degree of canal compromise and neurological deficit, as the neurological deficit is related to the initial injury and the canal compromise is related to the subsequent position of the bony fragments.

2. **a. With curves of 20–29°, 40% of patients who are Risser 0–1 are at risk of curve progression.**
This question tests the knowledge of curve progression according to the curve magnitude and maturity as assessed by the Risser sign. For curves of 20–29° in an immature child with a Risser sign of 0 or 1, the incidence of progression is 68%. Smaller curves (<19°) in an immature child (Risser 0–1), and larger curves (20–29°) in a mature child (Risser 2 or more) have an incidence of progression of 22% and 23% respectively.

3. **b. The sympathetic trunk, lying longitudinally along the lateral border of the psoas, is at risk during this procedure.**
The sympathetic trunk lies longitudinally along the medial border of the psoas. An injury to the sympathetic chain results in a warm and red foot on the ipsilateral side to the approach (left in this case), giving the appearance that the normal foot is cold and pale.

4. **e. Neurological deficit associated with compression from neurofibromata or kyphoscoliosis is uncommon.**
The typical curve in NF-1 is a dystrophic curve characterized by a short and sharp curvature. Other dystrophic features include scalloping of the vertebral bodies, enlargement of the neural foramina, marked rotation of the apical vertebra and pencilling of the ribs or transverse processes. Approximately 17% of patients with spinal deformity secondary to NF may have a neurological compromise due to tumour or deformity.

5. **b. This syndrome is also known as cast syndrome.**
Superior mesenteric artery syndrome also known as cast syndrome is an uncommon but well-recognized complication of scoliosis surgery. It occurs more commonly in thin female

Postgraduate Orthopaedics, ed. Kesavan Sri-Ram. Published by Cambridge University Press.
© Cambridge University Press 2012.

patients following correction of scoliosis by a cast or instrumentation. As a result of the curve correction, the angle between the SMA and the aorta is narrowed resulting in the compression of the third part of the duodenum. Initial treatment includes oral intake restriction, nasogastric suction and intravenous fluid administration. The majority of cases settle with conservative measures. In rare cases of failed non-operative treatment, surgical intervention is indicated.

6. **d. According to Waddell *et al*, non-organic signs should be equated with malingering or the presence of a psychological problem.**
Waddell's inappropriate/non-organic signs include: pain on axial compression and pelvic rotation, resisted hip flexion, non-dermatomal sensory loss, non-anatomical tenderness to light touch, cogwheel 'give way' weakness, straight leg rise (SLR) discrepancy and overreaction. The presence of more than three signs indicates non-organic features; however, the presence of the non-organic signs should not be equated with malingering but should alert the clinician to the need for more comprehensive testing.

7. **d. An ipsilateral far lateral disc herniation at L5–S1.**
A paracentral disc herniation at L4–L5 or a far lateral disc herniation at L5–S1 most commonly result in an L5 radiculopathy and therefore weakness of the gluteus medius, resulting in a Trendelenburg gait. A paracentral herniation at L5–S1 most commonly affects the S1 nerve root. A paracentral herniation at L3–L4 and a far lateral herniation at L4–L5 all affect the L4 root.

8. **a. It originates underneath the anterior longitudinal ligament and can cause destruction of several contiguous levels.**
Spinal tuberculosis (TB) originates in the metaphysis of the vertebral body and spreads under the anterior longitudinal ligament causing destruction of several contiguous levels and skip lesions in 15% of the cases. The disc spaces are preserved in the early stages of the infection, which differentiates TB of the spine from pyogenic infection. Contrary to a spinal cord injury occurring as a result of meningomyelitis, a cord injury secondary to direct pressure from the TB abscess or the bony sequestra carries a good prognosis.

9. **c. A space available for the cord (SAC) of less than 14 mm or an ADI of more than 9–10 mm is an indication for spinal stabilization.**
An atlantoaxial subluxation occurs in 60–80% of cases of rheumatoid arthritis (RA) as the result of pannus formation at the synovial joints between the dens and the ring of C1. An ADI of >3.5 mm on flexion extension is a common finding in RA and indicates instability; however, it is not necessarily an indication for surgery. A SAC <14 mm or an ADI >9–10 mm is associated with an increased risk of neurological injury and usually requires surgical intervention. A Ranawat C1–C2 index is the distance from the centre of the C2 pedicle to a line connecting the anterior and posterior arches of C1. It is the most reproducible measurement of invagination. A C1–C2 index <13 mm indicates basilar invagination. Subaxial subluxation occurs in 20% of cases of RA, a subluxation >4 mm or more than 20% of the body is indicative of cord compression.

10. **d. Right L5 perineural fibrosis.**
Gadolinium-enhanced MRI scans are helpful post discectomy in differentiating between recurrence of disc herniation, which does not enhance with gadolinium, and perineural

fibrosis, which shows enhancement around the root. A schwannoma enhances with gadolinium although the root would be enlarged. Systemically the patient is well and there is no evidence of fluid collection on scanning to suggest an infective process.

11. e. **Pain avoidance.**
Yellow flags are psychological factors shown to be indicative of long-term chronicity and disability which include a negative attitude that back pain is harmful or severely disabling resulting in fear avoidance behaviour and reduced activity levels. There is a tendency to depression, low morale and social withdrawal.

12. e. **Decompression of the syrinx in patients above the age of 10 years will improve or stabilize the scoliotic curve.**
Syringomyelia usually results from lesions that partially obstruct cerebrospinal fluid (CSF) flow including craniocervical junction abnormalities (Chiari malformations), spinal cord trauma and tumours. It often presents with central cord syndrome. Light touch, proprioception and vibration sensation are usually preserved. In most patients over the age of ten, surgical treatment of scoliosis is most likely necessary due to a large initial scoliosis curve or curve progression even after syrinx drainage.

13. c. **Complete spinal cord injury.**
An intact bulbocavernous reflex indicates that the patient is not in a state of spinal shock and therefore the cord injury can be classified as a complete injury pattern in this scenario.

14. b. **Complete C5.**
Spinal cord injury levels are defined by the ASIA classification. Complete injuries are defined as: No voluntary anal contraction with a distal power MRC 0 and 0/2 distal sensory score (absent perianal sensation) with an intact bulbocavernous reflex (patient not in spinal shock). This patient is functional at C5 (deltoid and biceps) and not functional at C6 (wrist extensors) and C7 (wrist flexion and triceps). His last functional level is C5 indicating a C5 neurological level. It is complete as his distal motor and sensory function is absent.

15. c. **Enlarged intervertebral foramina.**
Diastematomyelia is a congenital anomaly caused by a bony, cartilaginous or fibrous bar that results in the 'splitting' of the spinal cord in a sagittal direction. When the split does not reunite distally, the condition is referred to as diplomyelia. Diastematomyelia can lead to tethering of the cord and may be associated with neurological deficit. An intrapedicular widening is suggestive. An enlarged intervertebral foramina is seen in patients with neurofibroma.

16. a. **Left lateral foot numbness.**
A foraminal or extraforaminal/far lateral disc herniation affects the exiting root (in this case L5), whilst a paracentral or posterolateral disc herniation affects the traversing root (S1). An EHL and EDL weakness would be consistent with an L5 compression. Dorsomedial foot and lateral calf numbness would also be the result of an L5 compression.

17. c. **Infantile scoliosis commonly affects girls and is usually left-sided.**
Infantile scoliosis occurs between the ages of 2 months and 3 years. It commonly affects boys and is usually left-sided. An MRI scan should be performed in infantile scoliosis to

exclude a Chiari, syrinx or cord tethering. The term early onset scoliosis is now widely used and includes infantile, juvenile and any scoliosis that occurs before the age of 10 years.

18. c.   **Tension signs are usually positive.**
Central stenosis can be congenital or acquired. Acquired stenosis is the more common type occurring usually secondary to degenerative changes owing to enlargement of the osteoarthritic facets resulting in medial encroachment. It can also occur as the result of various disease processes such as Paget's disease. It is more common in men because their canal diameter is smaller at the L3–L5 levels than that of women. Tension signs are rarely positive. Unlike lateral recess stenosis or a herniated disc, a central stenosis does not commonly result in leg pain in a dermatomal distribution.

19. d.   **A posterior instrumentation should stop at the distal most tilted vertebra.**
Scheuermann's kyphosis is a kyphotic deformity of >45° in the thoracic spine with >5° anterior wedging across three consecutive vertebrae. The condition is often associated with a lumbar hyperlordosis. A mild scoliosis can sometimes be present. It is differentiated from postural kyphosis by the rigidity of the curve. It is the most common cause of thoracic back pain in older children and adolescents. An MRI scan is indicated to look for disc herniation, cord abnormalities and spinal stenosis. Surgery is indicated for curves >80° in skeletally mature patients, it entails a posterior spinal fusion with dual-rod instrumentation +/− anterior release and interbody fusion. The fusion level should stop distally at the vertebra which is parallel to the floor (usually the L3 level). A ligamentum flavum excision should be performed at the apex to prevent buckling of the ligament and therefore decrease the risk of neurological deficit.

20. a.   **With age, the proteoglycan (PG) synthesis decreases; however, the PG concentration increases due to the drop in the water content.**
The intervertebral disc is made up of the annulus fibrosis and nucleus pulposus. The annulus is rich in collage type I and resists tensile forces; the nucleus is rich in type II collagen and resists compressive forces. Age-related changes include:

- A decrease in proteoglycan synthesis resulting in an overall decrease in the proteoglycan concentration despite a drop in the water content.
- Chondroitin sulphate concentration decreases.
- The absolute quantity of collagen remains constant (there is a decrease in type I and increase in type III collagen).

21. b.   **The mechanism of injury is a primary hyperflexion of the neck.**
A hangman's fracture is a traumatic spondylolisthesis of C2 on C3 as a result of bilateral fracture of C2 pars or pedicles. The mechanism of injury is an extension injury (causes pars fracture) with a secondary flexion (disrupts the posterior longitudinal ligament (PLL) and the disc) resulting in the anterolisthesis. In 30% there is a concomitant C-spine fracture. There is usually no neurological deficit except in type III. Levine and Edwards have classified this fracture as follows:

Type I – minimal displacement and angulation with an intact disc. Treatment: Philadelphia-like collar.

Type II – displaced fracture of the pars with >3 mm displacement and significant angulation (disc and PLL disrupted). Reduce with traction then apply halo for 2 months.

Type IIA – no horizontal displacement but significant angulation. Reduction with hyperextension WITHOUT TRACTION then apply halo for 2 months.

Type III – is associated with bilateral facet dislocation and requires an open reduction of the dislocation with C2/C3 fusion.

22. **d.** **A ligamentous chance fracture should be treated using a compression construct with one level above and one level below the fracture**.
A chance fracture is the result of a flexion-distraction injury (seatbelt injury). It can be bony, ligamentous or mixed. Gastrointestinal injuries occur in 50% of cases. The bony lesions unite non–operatively with a brace in extension. The ligamentous type may remain unstable and therefore should be treated operatively using a compression construct (restore the tension band) with one level above and one level below the fracture. A chance fracture is seldom associated with a neurological deficit unless translation occurs.

23. **d.** **Flexion/extension of the C-spine is often reduced**.
Contrary to the common belief, the classic triad of low posterior hairline, short neck and reduced range of movement is seen in fewer than 50% of patients with Klippel–Feil syndrome. A Sprengel deformity is seen in 33% of cases, congenital scoliosis occurs in 60% and renal abnormalities is encountered in 33% of cases. Lateral side bending is usually limited whilst flexion/extension is often preserved.

24. **b.** **A disc and the vertebrae above and below, including their interlocking facet joints**.
A spinal motion segment is made up of a disc with its adjacent vertebrae and their interlocking facet joints devoid of musculature.

25. **d.** **Helical CT scan with a 2–3 mm slice from the base of the skull to at least T1**.
If it is anticipated that a patient will remain unconscious, unassessable or unreliable for clinical examination for more than 48 hours, radiological spinal clearance imaging should be undertaken. For the cervical spine, the appropriate standard is a thin-slice (2–3 mm) helical CT scan from the base of the skull to at least T1 with both sagittal and coronal reconstructions. This scan can demonstrate the subtle abnormalities offering high sensitivity and specificity in detecting unstable injuries of the cervical spine. Plain radiographs are insensitive in the neck and the upper thoracic spine. MRI scanning has high sensitivity but only moderate specificity and is logistically difficult for ITU patients.

26. **d.** **Medical management with non-steroidal anti-inflammatory drugs (NSAIDs) is a satisfactory treatment modality in this case**.
Bone scan is almost invariably positive in osteoid osteoma. The natural history of osteoid osteoma is for spontaneous resolution in 6–7 years so medical management with non-steroidal anti-inflammatory drugs (NSAIDs) is an option for some patients. As scoliosis resolves with resection/ablation in a child under 11 years of age, an operative intervention should be undertaken in this case.

27. **d.** **Anterior cervical decompression and fusion**.
This patient has myelopathic changes within the cord probably as a result of an anterior degenerative disc. The presence of a fixed kyphosis of >10° is a contraindication to a

posterior decompression +/− fusion. In addition, posterior procedures are ineffective in this case as the anterior compression on the cord will remain. The anterior approach provides direct access to the disc herniation and provides immediate and long-term stability to the motion segment.

28. **d.   Recurrent laryngeal nerve injury risk is lower at the lower C-spine levels (C6–C7).** The injury risk of the recurrent laryngeal nerve is higher at the lower C-spine (C6–C7) as it initially descends into the thorax within the carotid sheath, then it curves around the aortic arch and ascends back into the neck running between the trachea and oesophagus to supply the larynx. The nerves are usually safe as long as the retractors are placed underneath the longus colli muscles.

29. **d.   A type II rotator subluxation indicates an insufficiency of the transverse and alar ligaments.** Atlantoaxial rotatory instability can occur after trauma or spontaneously. It is associated with Morquio syndrome, spondyloepiphyseal dysplasia, Larsen's syndrome, achondroplasia and Grisel's syndrome. It is present in 25% of children with Down syndrome. In type I, the odontoid acts as a pivot point and there is no anterior subluxation. In type II, one facet acts as a pivot with an ADI 3–5 mm. The transverse ligament is insufficient. In type III, the alar and transverse ligaments are incompetent resulting in bilateral facet subluxation with an ADI >5 mm.

30. **c.   A hyperextension injury in a patient with a facet joint hypertrophy and thickened ligamentum flavum.** Central cord syndrome is the most common incomplete spinal cord lesion. It is usually seen in patients with cervical spondylosis who sustain a hyperextension injury. The mechanism causes compression of the cord by osteophytes anteriorly and ligamentum flavum posteriorly.

EMQs

1. **1. a. Central cord syndrome.** 2. **c. Brown-Séquard syndrome.** 3. **b. Anterior cord syndrome.**

Central cord syndrome is the most common incomplete spinal cord injury presenting with greater loss of neurons in the upper extremities than in the lower ones. It has an overall fair prognosis. Brown-Séquard syndrome occurs as a result of penetrating trauma resulting in ipsilateral proprioception loss and motor weakness with loss of contralateral pain and temperature sensation. An anterior cord syndrome is related to vascular insufficiency of the anterior two-thirds of the cord resulting in loss of power and pain with preserved proprioception and vibration sense. It carries the worst prognosis among the incomplete spinal cord injuries.

2. **1. d. Right far lateral L4/L5 disc herniation.** 2. **c. Right paracentral L4/L5 disc herniation.** 3. **f. Right posterolateral L5/S1 disc herniation.**

Posterolateral or paracentral discs are the most common type occurring in approximately 90–95% of cases. The most common location is L4/L5 followed by L5/S1. Foraminal and far lateral discs occur in 5–10% of the cases. A posterolateral/paracentral disc affects the lower, traversing nerve root (L5 root at the L4/L5 level). A foraminal/far lateral disc affects the upper, exiting root (L5 at the L5/S1 level). A paraspinal approach (Wiltse) is indicated for far lateral disc herniation.

3. **1. a. Dysplastic.** 2. **d. Degenerative at L4/L5.** 3. **c. Isthmic type IIB.**

Dysplastic spondylolisthesis (Wiltse-Newman type I) occurs secondary to congenital abnormalities of the lumbosacral articulation (malorientated or hypoplastic facets (scenario 1), sacral deficiency or poorly developed pars). Spondylolysis is not a feature of the dysplastic type. An isthmic spondylolisthesis (Wiltse type II) describes a defect in the pars interarticularis as a result of repetitive hyperextension and is the most common type in the paediatric population. It is subdivided into three subtypes:

Type IIA – disruption of the pars as a result of a fatigue fracture.

Type IIB – elongation of the pars without disruption (scenario 3).

Type IIC – acute fracture through the pars.

It is important to note that an isthmic spondylolisthesis at L5/S1 causes a compression of the L5 exiting root. Compression may involve the hypertrophic fibrous repair tissue at the pars defect. A degenerative spondylolisthesis is more common in diabetic females above 40 years of age. It occurs most often at the L4/L5 level and results in central or lateral recess stenosis affecting therefore the traversing/descending root (L5 in an L4/L5 degenerative spondylolisthesis, scenario 2).

4. **1. c. C6.** 2. **d. C7.** 3. **c. C6.**

A functional level in a patient with spinal cord injury is determined by the most distal sensory and motor level at which most of the muscles at that level have a fair motor grade. Patients at C5 can use a motorized wheelchair with hand control. Patients at C6 have a much better function than C5 due to the ability to bring their hands to the mouth and feed themselves (wrist extension and supination intact with absent wrist flexion). They have improved manual wheelchair function, can drive a car with manual controls and have an independent mobility (scenarios 1 and 3). Patients at C7 have improved triceps strength and can cut meat.

5. **1. e. Eosinophilic granuloma.** 2. **d. Haemangioma.** 3. **f. Giant cell tumour.**
Eosinophilic granuloma is usually seen in children younger than 10 years. It is often present in the thoracic spine and is associated with progressive back pain. It classically results in vertebral flattening (vertebra plana). The classic patient with haemangioma has jailhouse striations on plain radiographs and spikes of bone on CT. Giant cell tumour is usually seen in the fourth and fifth decade. It destroys the vertebral body in an expansile fashion. The recommended treatment is surgical excision and bone grafting. A high recurrence rate is reported.

6. **1. g. CT-guided radiofrequency ablation therapy.** 2. **c. Chemotherapy +/− local radiation.** 3. **f. Wide-margin surgical resection +/− radiotherapy.**
In the first scenario, the nidus measures <1.5 cm suggesting most likely the diagnosis of an osteoid osteoma rather than an osteoblastoma. Failure of conservative treatment would necessitate an intervention. If the lesion is accessible through CT guidance then radiofrequency ablation can be considered. Ivory vertebrae and small round cell infiltrate are suggestive of lymphoma. Non-operative multi-agent chemotherapy +/− local irradiation is the mainstay of treatment. Radiation may be added to obtain local control in the area of the lesion. The last clinical scenario is a case of chordoma. Treatment is operative with wide-margin surgical resection often requiring to sacrifice the sacral nerve roots. Local recurrence is common and therefore radiation is often added if the margins are not achieved.

7. **1. b. Cauda equina syndrome.** 2. **f. Vascular claudication.** 3. **g. Spinal stenosis.**
The first scenario is a classic case of acute cauda equina syndrome, including saddle anaesthesia and urinary retention with a significant residual urine volume. Patients with vascular claudication have usually a fixed claudication distance with pain described as cramp or tightness in the calf (distal-proximal pain). Pain is brought on by walking uphill or riding a bicycle and relieved by standing erect or lying flat. Patients with neurogenic claudication have a variable claudication distance with proximal-distal pain. Patients must sit or get in a flexed position for relief of pain.

8. **1. f. Flexion 'teardrop' fracture.** 2. **a. Jefferson's fracture.** 3. **g. Unilateral facet dislocation.**
The flexion teardrop fracture is the most severe injury of the cervical spine. It results from a combination of extreme flexion and compressive forces. It commonly results from a dive in a shallow pool of water. It often presents with quadriplegia and loss of anterior column sensation. Jefferson fracture is classically described as a four-part burst fracture of the atlas with combined anterior and posterior arch fractures. It occurs as a result of axial compression and has a low rate of neurological deficit due to the large breadth of C1 canal. In the last scenario the bow tie sign is a classic for a unilateral facet dislocation, where a forward rotation of one side occurs around the other fixed side. The body subluxes forward by 25% of the anteroposterior diameter. The lateral masses of the displaced vertebra overlap on the lateral view giving the bow tie sign.

9. **1. c. Posterior instrumented fusion of the thoracic curve.** 2. **a. Boston brace.** 3. **g. Spinal fusion down to pelvis.**
The first case scenario tests the knowledge of the definition of a structural curve (bending Cobb angle >25°). In this case the thoracic curve is structural (does not correct to <25°)

whilst the lumbar curve corrects to $18°$ indicating its non-structural characteristic; therefore, a posterior thoracic fusion is a viable treatment option. In the second scenario, the patient is still premenarchal with $<45°$ curve. It would therefore be reasonable to treat this patient with a Boston brace as the apex is below T8. In the last scenario, patients with neuromuscular scoliosis, who are wheelchair users, with worsening sitting balance should be treated with a posterior instrumentation down to the pelvis.

10. 1. **c. Diffuse idiopathic skeletal hyperostosis (DISH). 2. g. Destructive spondyloarthropathy 3. b. Ankylosing spondylitis.**
DISH, also known as Forestier disease, is defined by the presence of non-marginal osteophytes at three successive levels (differentiated from ankylosing spondylitis, which has vertical or marginal osteophytes). Destructive spondyloarthropathy is seen in haemodialysis patients with chronic renal failure, it typically involves three adjacent vertebrae and their intervening disc spaces. The process may resemble infection.

11. 1. **g. L4. 2. h. L5. 3. i. S1.**
The lower nerve roots are summarized below:

Nerve root	Motor	Sensory	Reflex
L1	Hip flexion	Groin	None
L2	Hip flexion	Outer thigh	None
L3	Knee extension	Knee	None
L4	Ankle dorsiflexion	Inner leg	Knee jerk
L5	Big toe extension	Big toe	None
S1	Ankle plantarflexion	Lateral foot	Ankle jerk
S2	Knee flexion	Back of the knee	None

12. 1. **g. Pavlov. 2. c. Space available for the cord (SAC). 3. b. Ranawat.**
The Pavlov (or Torg) ratio is the canal:vertebral body width, and should be 1. A value less than 0.80 is considered a risk factor for neurological injury after minor trauma such as hyperextension. A number of radiological lines and spaces are used when assessing a rheumatoid cervical spine and relate to atlantoaxial subluxation and cranial settling (or basilar invagination). They include:

- Atlantodens interval (ADI) – this is assessed on both flexion and extension views; instability is present when there is a 3.5 mm difference on each view; a 7 mm difference suggests disruption of the alar ligaments; a difference of more than 9 mm is associated with an increase in neurological injury.
- Space available for the cord (SAC) – this is the posterior space and a distance of less than 14 mm is considered a risk factor for neurological injury.
- Ranawat's line is from the centre of the C2 pedicle to the C1 arch and is normally 17 mm; a distance less than 13 mm would suggest cranial settling.
- McRae's line is the foramen magnum line drawn from the anterior margin of the foramen to the posterior margin and the tip of the dens should not cross this line.

- Chamberlain's line is from the posterior end of the hard palate to the posterior lip of the foramen magnum and normally the tip of the dens is no more than 3 mm above this line.
- McGregor's line is from the hard palate to the posterior occipit curve and normally the tip of the dens would be more than 8 mm above this line in men and more than 10 mm in women.
- Wackenheim line (clivus line) is a line extended inferiorly from the clivus and should pass through the dens of the axis or be tangential to it.

13. 1. b. Lateral spinothalamic tract. 2. f. Dorsal spinocerebellar tract. 3. d. Lateral corticospinal tract.
There are many tracts in the spinal cord. The ascending (sensory) tracts include the dorsal column (deep touch, proprioception and vibration), lateral spinothalamic tract (pain and temperature) and anterior spinothalamic tract (light touch). The descending (motor) tracts include the lateral corticospinal tract (motor control of ipsilateral limbs) and ventral corticospinal tract (motor control of central axial and girdle muscles). The spinocerebellar tracts are involved in propioception, coordination of posture and movement of individual muscles of lower extremities. The information is obtained from muscle spindles (dorsal) and Golgi tendon organs (ventral).

14. 1. l. Bowstring test. 2. e. Lhermitte's sign. 3. c. Hoffman's test.
The bowstring test is performed after a positive straight leg raise is elicited; the angle of hip elevation is decreased to decrease the radicular pain and then pressure is applied to the popliteal fossa, over the nerve, to reproduce symptoms. Lhermitte's sign is an electric shock-like sensation shooting down the spine when flexing the cervical spine. Hoffman's test involves quickly snapping or flicking the middle fingernail; if positive, the tip of the index finger, ring finger, and/or thumb suddenly flex in response, and this indicates cervical myelopathy.

15. 1. f. 20%. 2. b. 0–1%. 3. g. 30%.
In general practice, the overall incidence of herniated nucleus pulposus in patients who have new onset lower back pain is less than 2%. However, incidence of lumbar herniated nucleus pulposus in asymptomatic patients less than 60 years of age is between 20% and 25%. Following scoliosis surgery, the risk of neurological injury has been reported as 0.8%. Concomitant spinal injury is common after particular cervical injuries. The risk of concomitant cervical injury after hangman's fractures is 30% and the risk of concomitant spinal injury after C1 fracture is 50%.

Selected references

American Spinal Injury Association. *International Standards for Neurological and Functional Classification of Spinal Cord Injury Patients*. Chicago, IL, 2000.

Andersson GB, Deyo RA. History and physical examination in patients with herniated lumbar discs. *Spine* 1996; **21**: 10S–18S.

BOA. BOAST2: *Spinal Clearance in the Trauma Patient*. 2008.

Boos N, Weissbach S, Rohrbach H *et al.* Classification of age-related changes in the intervertebral discs. *Spine (Phila PA 1976)* 2002; **27**(23): 2631–44.

Chance GQ. Note on a type of flexion fracture of the spine. *Br J Radiol* 1948; **21**: 452–3.

Hensinger RN, Lang JE, MacEwenGO. Klippel-Feil syndrome: a constellation of the associated anomalies. *JBJS Am* 1974; (**56**): 1246–53.

Herkowitz HN, Kurz LT, Overholt DP. Surgical management of cervical soft disc herniation. A comparison between the anterior and posterior approach. *Spine(Phila PA 1976)* 1990; **15**(10): 1026–30.

Hoppenfeld S, deBoer P, Buckley R. *Surgical Exposures in Orthopaedics: The Anatomic Approach*, 3rd edn. Philadelphia, Lippincott Williams and Wilkins, 2009.

Levine AM, Edwards CC. The management of traumatic spondylolisthesis of the axis. *J Bone Joint Surg Am* 1985; **67**: 217–26.

Lonstein JE, Carlson JM. The prediction of curve progression in untreated idiopathic scoliosis during growth. *J Bone Joint Surg Am* 1984; **66**: 1061–71.

Miller MD. *Review of Orthopaedics*, 5th edn. Philadelphia, Elsevier, 2008.

Rhee JM, Shaufele M, Abud WA. Radiculopathy and the herniated lumbar disc. *J Bone Joint Surg Am* 2006; **88**: 2070–81.

Tribus CB. Scheuermann's kyphosis in adolescents and adults: diagnosis and management. *J Am Acad Orthop Surg* 1998; **6**: 36–43.

Waddell G, McCulloh JA, Kummel E, Venner RM. Nonorganic physical signs in low-back pain. *Spine (Phila Pa 1976)* 1980; **5**: 117–25.

Winter RB, Moe JH, Bradford DS *et al.* Spine deformity in neurofibromatosis. *J Bone Joint Surg Am* 1979; **61**: 677–94.

Yeom JS, Lee CK, Park KW *et al.* Scoliosis associated with syringomyelia: analysis of MRI and curve progression. *Eur Spine J* 2007; **16**(10): 1629–35.

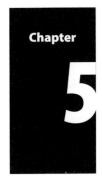

Hip and pelvis: Questions

Nashat Siddiqui and Phil Kerr

MCQs

1. **If surgery for intracapsular fracture fixation is not carried out within 12 hours, avascular necrosis (AVN) and non-union rates are affected in this way?**
   a. No difference between AVN and non-union rates.
   b. AVN higher, no change in non-union.
   c. No change in AVN, non-union higher.
   d. AVN and non-union both higher.
   e. AVN higher but non-union lower.

2. **Injury to which artery is most likely to cause uncontrollable bleeding during the posterior approach to the hip?**
   a. Inferior gluteal.
   b. Superior gluteal.
   c. Pudendal.
   d. Ascending branch of lateral circumflex femoral.
   e. Popliteal.

3. **With regard to closed suction drains used in surgery, which of the following is true?**
   a. Wound infection is higher with use of drains.
   b. Haematoma formation is lower with use of drains.
   c. Wound dehiscence is more likely without the use of drains.
   d. Blood transfusion is more likely with the use of drains.
   e. Bruising is more likely with the use of drains.

4. **What is the predominant source of femoral head perfusion?**
   a. Lateral circumflex artery.
   b. Obturator artery.
   c. Medial circumflex artery.
   d. Descending branch of lateral circumflex artery.
   e. Superior gluteal artery.

5. **The main internal rotators of the hip are?**
   a. Gluteus minimus and tensor fascia lata.
   b. Obturator internus, superior and inferior gemelli.

Postgraduate Orthopaedics, ed. Kesavan Sri-Ram. Published by Cambridge University Press.

   c. Iliopsoas.

   d. Piriformis and quadratus femoris.

   e. Piriformis and gluteus medius.

6. **In Judet views of the pelvis, the right obturator oblique view shows?**

   a. Pubic symphysis in the centre of the obturator foramen.

   b. Posterior wall and anterior column of the right acetabulum.

   c. Anterior wall and posterior column of the right acetabulum.

   d. The right obturator foramen perpendicular to the plane of the X-ray cassette.

   e. The sacroiliac joint on the right side even if a c-clamp is applied.

7. **Core decompression following avascular necrosis (AVN) of the femoral head is more likely to be successful if the patient has not progressed beyond?**

   a. FICAT I.

   b. FICAT II.

   c. FICAT III.

   d. FICAT IV.

   e. FICAT V.

8. **In which situation following deep infection of a total hip replacement could single-stage revision be considered?**

   a. The erythrocyte sedimentation rate (ESR) and C-reactive protein (CRP) are not raised.

   b. It is less than 6 months since primary surgery.

   c. There is a known organism from preoperative aspirate and the patient has commenced antibiotics.

   d. The organism is seen and identified via fresh frozen specimen sent during surgery, and the patient is commenced on antibiotics.

   e. The infected implants were cemented with antibiotic-loaded cement.

9. **In planning total hip replacement for a patient with Paget's disease, which of the following is not an expected finding?**

   a. Acetabular protrusion.

   b. Higher than usual blood loss.

   c. Harder than usual bone.

   d. Valgus deformity of femoral neck.

   e. High cardiac output.

10. **The following are known causes of sciatic nerve dysfunction following total hip replacement except?**

   a. Post-operative haematoma (e.g. subgluteal) around the sciatic nerve.

   b. Limb lengthening over 5 cm.

   c. Direct laceration during surgery.

   d. Tissue trauma during surgery from retractors.

   e. Pressure from straps of abduction wedge pillow.

11. **Which of the following is true regarding labral tears of the acetabulum?**
    a. They are frequently caused by femoral head osteophytes.
    b. They result in lack of external rotation of the hip during normal gait.
    c. They predispose to early osteoarthritic change.
    d. They are associated with degenerate changes and cysts when due to femoro-acetabular impingement.
    e. They are most commonly seen after posterior hip dislocation.

12. **For infection following total hip replacement, wound washout and exchange of accessible components is acceptable management if?**
    a. Infection is within 3 weeks of surgery.
    b. Known organism is cultured from hip aspirate.
    c. Patient cannot tolerate general anaesthetic.
    d. Ceramic head and liner *in situ*.
    e. Infection greater than 12 but less than 36 months from surgery.

13. **Which of the following is not one of the trabecular patterns in the proximal femur?**
    a. Greater trochanter group.
    b. Lesser trochanter group.
    c. Principle compressive group.
    d. Secondary compressive group.
    e. Principle tensile group.

14. **What is meralgia paraesthetica due to?**
    a. Compression of the obturator nerve at the obturator foramen.
    b. Haematoma around part of the sciatic nerve.
    c. Compression of the lateral cutaneous nerve of thigh.
    d. Compression of the femoral nerve (e.g. by a weightlifter's belt).
    e. Diabetes.

15. **Which of the following is the greatest risk factor for heterotopic ossification following elective total hip replacement?**
    a. Previous formation of heterotopic ossification.
    b. Hypercalcaemia.
    c. Male.
    d. Head injury within the previous 48 hours.
    e. Inflamed greater trochanteric bursa.

16. **A patient is to have primary total hip replacement and takes methotrexate for rheumatoid arthritis. Methotrexate should be?**
    a. Stopped 24 hours before surgery.
    b. Stopped 1 week before surgery.
    c. Reduced to half the dose but not stopped.
    d. Continued as usual.
    e. Gradually reduced to stop 24 hours before surgery and then restarted 2 weeks following surgery.

17. A 72-year-old patient is suspected to have an infected total hip replacement, rather than aseptic loosening, 8 years following surgery. Which of the following would be a useful investigation to differentiate between them?
    a. Radio-labelled white cell scan.
    b. Radionuclide bone scan.
    c. Plain X-ray.
    d. Hip aspiration.
    e. Ultrasound scan of the hip joint.

18. Which of the following is true regarding impaction grafting for revision total hip replacement with femoral bone loss?
    a. It is best with a polished tapered stem.
    b. It should subside less than 2 mm in the first year in order to predict successful outcome.
    c. If subsiding more than 2 mm after the first year, it should be considered for early revision.
    d. It is designed for use with uncemented stems.
    e. It is associated with a significantly higher rate of deep infection due to the large amount of allograft used.

19. What is the effect of repairing the posterior capsule in the posterior approach for total hip replacement?
    a. Reduce dislocation by 20%.
    b. Reduce dislocation by a magnitude of 10.
    c. Reduce dislocation by 100%.
    d. No effect on dislocation rate.
    e. No longer recommended for posterior approach to the hip.

20. Which of the following is the most important prognostic indicator for the success of a hydroxyapatite (HA)-coated stem?
    a. Pore size.
    b. Coating of at least 50% of the stem.
    c. Pore density.
    d. Pore depth.
    e. Thickness of HA of at least 50 μm.

21. A 27-year-old patient presents with groin pain and clicking. He has a history of mild developmental dysplasia of the hip (DDH) as a child. Which of the following is the most likely finding on a plain radiograph?
    a. Acetabular osteophyte.
    b. Acetabular cyst.
    c. Femoral head subarticular cysts.
    d. Femoral head/neck junction prominence.
    e. Femoral neck stress fracture.

22. A 74-year-old patient has developed degenerate change in her hip requiring total hip replacement. She has previously had a pertrochanteric femoral fracture fixed with a dynamic hip screw device. What is the correct surgical management?
    a. Do not perform total hip replacement due to poor outcome.

b. Remove metalwork, use strut allograft and cable plate to reinforce femur, then use fully coated uncemented stem.

c. Remove the sliding screw only, and perform hip resurfacing to prevent risk of diaphyseal fracture.

d. Remove metalwork, use strut allograft and cable plate to reinforce femur, then use cemented stem.

e. Remove metalwork, insert cemented stem passing two cortical thicknesses below lowest screw hole.

23. **Following total hip replacement, deep infection is?**
    a. Less in ceramic than polyethylene cups.
    b. The same for ceramic and polyethylene cups.
    c. More in ceramic than polyethylene cups.
    d. More with the anterior approach.
    e. More with the posterior approach.

24. **Which of the following is true of the centre-edge angle of Wiberg?**
    a. It is only useful until the age of 12 months.
    b. If greater than 15°, it is normal.
    c. It is the angle made between Hilgenreiner's line and the roof of the acetabulum.
    d. If less than 15°, it is one of the indications for pelvic osteotomy.
    e. It cannot be measured once the triradiate cartilage has ossified.

25. **A 40-year-old patient is developing avascular necrosis of the femoral head. The contour is normal (i.e. no collapse), although structural changes are evident on MRI. What is the preferred treatment?**
    a. Hip resurfacing arthroplasty.
    b. Non-vascularized fibular graft.
    c. Low dose steroid for 18 weeks.
    d. Core decompression.
    e. Vascularized fibular graft.

26. **Which nerve is at risk during the ilio-inguinal approach to the pelvis, and often needs to be divided?**
    a. Anterior cutaneous branch of femoral nerve.
    b. Posterior branch of obturator nerve.
    c. Lateral cutaneous nerve of thigh.
    d. Anterior branch of obturator nerve.
    e. Cutaneous branch of obturator nerve.

27. **What type of lubrication is found in hard-on-hard total hip replacements at the point when the two articulating surfaces are not in contact?**
    a. Boundary.
    b. Boosted.
    c. Squeeze film.
    d. Elastohydrodynamic.
    e. Hydrodynamic.

28. **When cementing a femoral stem, what is thought to be the most likely cause for severe hypotension related to 'bone cement implantation syndrome' (BCIS)?**
    a. Anaphylaxis to polymethylmethacrylate (PMMA) molecules.
    b. Multiple emboli.
    c. Exothermic effect of cement temperature.
    d. Metabolites of the monomer entering the circulation causing vasodilatation.
    e. Large surface area in femoral medullary cavity to absorb methylmethacrylate monomer, as opposed to small area in acetabulum.

29. **In the posterior thigh, the sciatic nerve lies between which two muscles?**
    a. Gluteus maximus and biceps femoris.
    b. Gluteus maximus and piriformis.
    c. Gluteus maximus and adductor magnus.
    d. Superior gemellus and obturator internus.
    e. Superior gemellus and inferior gemellus.

30. **Which type of pelvic injury is most likely to result in urethral/bladder injury?**
    a. Vertical shear >2 cm.
    b. Lateral compression.
    c. Bilateral obturator ring fractures.
    d. Anterior pelvic arch displaced >1 cm.
    e. Inwardly displaced parasymphyseal fracture >1 cm.

EMQs

1. **Surgical approaches to the pelvis**
   a. Sartorius and tensor fascia lata
   b. Internal oblique
   c. Rectus femoris and sartorius
   d. Gluteus maximus and gluteus medius
   e. Posterior division of obturator nerve
   f. Inguinal ligament
   g. Inferior gluteal
   h. Adductor brevis and adductor magnus
   i. Rectus abdominis

From the list of options above, choose the most appropriate option for each of the following statements. Each option may be used once, more than once or not at all.
   1. These muscles are elevated in the Kocher–Langenbeck approach to the acetabulum.
   2. In the anterior approach to the pubic symphysis these muscles are divided but not denervated.
   3. This structure may be damaged if the anterior superior iliac spine is taken during bone graft harvesting.

2. **Radiological loosening of total hip replacement implants**
   a. 1, 2, 3
   b. 1 to 7 inclusive
   c. 1, 3
   d. 7, 8, 9
   e. 6, 7
   f. 1, 2
   g. 3, 4, 5
   h. 4, 5

From the list of options above, choose the most appropriate option for each of the following statements. Each option may be used once, more than once or not at all.
   1. Delee and Charnley zones indicating total loosening of acetabular prosthesis.
   2. Gruen zones indicating calcar loosening of the stem.
   3. Gruen zones indicating distal loosening of the stem.

3. **Pelvic osteotomies**
   a. Ganz
   b. Shantz
   c. Pemberton
   d. Innominate/triple
   e. Salter
   f. Steel
   g. Chiari
   h. Shelf

From the list of options above, choose the most appropriate option for each of the following statements. Each option may be used once, more than once or not at all.
1. Relies on formation of fibrocartilage under the new acetabular roof.
2. Layers of bone graft used to build up deficient lateral acetabulum.
3. Osteotomies close to the acetabulum to redirect the orientation of the acetabulum.

4. **Position of hip arthrodesis**
   a. 15°
   b. 25–30°
   c. 0–5°
   d. 5–10°
   e. 50°
   f. 75°
   g. 100°
   h. 35°

From the list of options above, choose the most appropriate option for each of the following scenarios. Each option may be used once, more than once or not at all.
1. The desired position of flexion.
2. The desired position of adduction.
3. The desired position of internal/external rotation.

5. **Modes of hip failure and zones involved**
   a. Pistoning: stem and cement within bone
   b. Medial midstem pivot
   c. Calcar pivot
   d. Pistoning: stem within cement
   e. Bending cantilever
   f. Crevice corrosion
   g. Fretting corrosion
   h. Fatigue wear

From the list of options above, choose the most appropriate option for each of the following scenarios. Each option may be used once, more than once or not at all.
1. This is likely to result in most of the osteolysis in zones 4 and 5.
2. This is likely to result in most osteolysis in zones 1 and 2 and 6 and 7.
3. This is likely to show osteolysis in all seven zones.

6. **Avulsions from the pelvis**
   a. Gluteus maximus
   b. Gluteus medius
   c. Gluteus minimus
   d. Gracilis
   e. Rectus femoris
   f. Hamstrings
   g. Iliopsoas
   h. Adductor magnus

   i. Adductor longus
   j. Sartorius

From the list of options above, choose the most appropriate option for each of the following scenarios. Each option may be used once, more than once or not at all.
1. The muscle which causes an avulsion from the anterior inferior iliac spine.
2. The muscle which causes an avulsion from the ischial tuberosity.
3. The muscle which causes an avulsion from the anterior superior iliac spine.

7. Femoral neck stress fractures
   a. Total hip replacement
   b. Non-weight-bearing for 8 weeks
   c. Non-weight-bearing for 2 weeks, then gradual increase in weight-bearing
   d. Fully weight-bear with crutch assistance for 6 weeks
   e. Urgent/semi-elective internal fixation
   f. Emergency internal fixation
   g. Simple analgesia and reassurance
   h. Activity avoidance for 9 months
   i. Core decompression

From the list of options above, choose the most appropriate option for each of the following scenarios. Each option may be used once, more than once or not at all.
1. A keen 22-year-old amateur marathon runner with a superior femoral neck stress fracture and marked groin pain.
2. A keen 22-year-old amateur marathon runner with an inferior femoral neck stress fracture and moderate groin pain.
3. A 36-year-old who plays sport occasionally with an inferior femoral neck stress fracture and moderate groin pain.

8. Injuries around the hip
   a. Stress fracture of femoral neck
   b. Adductor strain
   c. Iliotibial band syndrome
   d. Labral tear
   e. Hip dislocation
   f. Hamstring avulsion
   g. Meralgia paraesthetica
   h. Greater trochanteric bursitis
   i. Avascular necrosis

From the list of options above, choose the most appropriate option for each of the following scenarios. Each option may be used once, more than once or not at all.
1. A 25-year-old male presents with groin pain and clicking, with no history of trauma.
2. A 19-year-old sprinter collapsed during a race, and has diffuse buttock pain.
3. A 22-year-old female long distance runner describes her hip as 'repeatedly dislocating' with lateral pain around the greater trochanter.

9. Evolution of cementing techniques
  a. Porosity reduction using a vacuum
  b. Antibiotic impregnated
  c. Tapered polished stem
  d. Finger packing
  e. Chlorophyll addition
  f. Pulsatile lavage
  g. Collarless stem
  h. Carbon dioxide jet preparation of femur

From the list of options above, choose the most appropriate option for each of the following scenarios. Each option may be used once, more than once or not at all.
  1. This is typically a third generation cementing technique.
  2. This is typically a second generation cementing technique.
  3. This is typically a first generation cementing technique.

10. Tumours around the pelvis
  a. Chondrosarcoma
  b. Ewing's sarcoma
  c. Giant cell tumour
  d. Enchondroma
  e. Osteochondroma
  f. Osteoid osteoma
  g. Synovial sarcoma
  h. Chordoma
  i. Adamantinoma

From the list of options above, choose the most appropriate option for each of the following scenarios. Each option may be used once, more than once or not at all.
  1. A 51-year-old patient complains of low back pain radiating to the left hip. Plain X-rays are suggestive of expansion of the sacrum, and the vertebrae may be involved. Histology shows vacuolated, physaliferous cells.
  2. A 60-year-old male with an enlarging mass on one side of his pelvis, which is bony with a firm soft tissue swelling overlying it. X-ray shows bone destruction with a mineralized pattern. Histology shows large cartilage cells often multinucleate.
  3. A 15-year-old girl with pain in the right iliac wing, fever, raised erythrocyte sedimentation rate (ESR) and white blood cell count. Histology shows small round cells.

11. Hip bearing surfaces
  a. Cobalt-chrome socket
  b. Cobalt-chrome acetabular shell with ceramic liner
  c. Polyethylene socket
  d. Cobalt-chrome acetabular shell with polyethylene liner
  e. Stainless steel acetabular shell with polyethylene liner
  f. Cobalt-chrome head
  g. Stainless steel head
  h. Titanium head

From the list of options above, choose the most appropriate option for each of the
following scenarios. Each option may be used once, more than once or not at all.
1. This component or combination has the highest wear rate when used as a bearing
   surface.
2. This component or combination is associated with 'stripe wear'.
3. This component or combination has the lowest 10-year revision rate when used in
   the acetabulum.

12. **A patient undergoes hip arthrodesis**
    a. 0–5%
    b. 20–30%
    c. 50–60%
    d. 40–50%
    e. 90–100%

From the list of options above, choose the most appropriate option for each of the
following scenarios. Each option may be used once, more than once or not at all.
1. The proportion of patients that can be expected to experience significant back pain.
2. The proportion of patients that can be expected to experience significant ipsilateral
   knee pain.
3. The proportion of patients that can be expected to experience significant
   contralateral hip pain.

13. **Organisms responsible for infected total hip replacements**
    a. Methicillin-resistant *Staphylococcus aureus* (MRSA)
    b. *Escherichia coli*
    c. Methicillin-sensitive *Staphylococcus aureus*
    d. *Salmonella*
    e. *Enterococcus*
    f. Streptococci
    g. Coagulase-negative staphylococcus
    h. *Klebsiella*
    i. *Acinetobacter*
    j. *Pseudomonas*

From the list of options above, choose the most appropriate option for each of the
following scenarios. Each option may be used once, more than once or not at all.
1. The commonest infecting organism in total hip replacements.
2. The second commonest infecting organism in total hip replacements.
3. The third commonest infecting organism in total hip replacements.

14. **Surgical approaches to the hip**
    a. Gracilis and adductor longus
    b. Gluteus maximus and gluteus medius
    c. Gluteus medius and tensor fascia lata
    d. Vastus lateralis and tensor fascia lata
    e. Gluteus maximus and short external rotators

    f.   Posterior division of obturator nerve
    g. Lateral cutaneous nerve of thigh
    h. Femoral nerve
    i.   Anterior division of obturator nerve

From the list of options above, choose the most appropriate option for each of the following questions. Each option may be used once, more than once or not at all.
1. The nerve in jeopardy with the medial (Ludloff) approach to the hip.
2. The muscle interval which is utilized in superficial dissection in the medial (Ludloff) approach to the hip.
3. The internervous plane which is utilized in the anterolateral (Watson-Jones) approach to the hip.

15. **Cementless fixation of implants**
    a. 10 μm
    b. 30 μm
    c. 50 μm
    d. 100 μm
    e. 150 μm
    f.   500 μm
    g. 40%
    h. 0.50%
    i.   1%

From the list of options above, choose the most appropriate option for each of the following questions. Each option may be used once, more than once or not at all.
1. With a porous coated surface, this is the minimum pore size for optimal fixation.
2. The maximum gap between implant and bone to allow ingrowth/ongrowth.
3. The maximum amount of micromotion allowed.

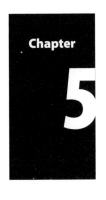

Chapter

5

Hip and pelvis: Answers

Nashat Siddiqui and Phil Kerr

MCQs

1. **a. No difference between AVN and non-union rates.**
Although it is common to treat these fractures with some urgency, a meta-analysis of 18 studies (564 fractures) showed no difference in these rates if surgery is carried out before or after 12 hours. A further study has shown no difference before or after 48 hours.

2. **a. Inferior gluteal.**
The inferior gluteal artery may retract into the pelvis, requiring the patient to be positioned supine and urgent laparotomy to tie off the internal iliac artery.

3. **d. Blood transfusion is more likely with the use of drains.**
In a Cochrane review of 36 studies (5697 surgical wounds), no statistically significant difference was found in the occurrence of infection, haematoma, dehiscence, or re-operation between patients with or without suction drains. Those with drains had a higher rate of transfusion, but lower rate of wound dressing reinforcement and bruising.

4. **c. Medial circumflex artery.**
The medial circumflex artery is a branch of the profunda femoris, originating from the external iliac. The blood supply is via subsynovial retinacular artery. The remainder is supplied by the artery of ligamentum teres (obturator artery) and lateral circumflex artery (profunda femoris).

5. **a. Gluteus minimus and tensor fascia lata.**
Gluteus minimus inserts anteriorly on the tip of greater trochanter, but gluteus medius inserts more posteriorly and therefore is more of an external rotator than minimus. Piriformis is, of course, an external rotator. Tensor fascia lata originates from the iliac crest and anterior superior iliac spine (ASIS) and via its attachment to the iliotibial band, acts as an internal rotator, abductor and flexor of the hip. Iliopsoas, which attaches to the lesser trochanter, is primarily a flexor of the hip. Although it is responsible for the externally rotated position of the femur in patients with femoral neck fractures, thereby acting as an external rotator of the hip, it does not have any significant rotational contribution in the uninjured femur.

6. **b. Posterior wall and anterior column of the right acetabulum.**
Judet views of the pelvis are: Obturator oblique, where the obturator foramen on that side is parallel to the X-ray cassette, by elevating the pelvis on that side, and shows the posterior wall and

Postgraduate Orthopaedics, ed. Kesavan Sri-Ram. Published by Cambridge University Press.
© Cambridge University Press 2012.

anterior column of the elevated acetabulum (mnemonic: OOPWAC – Obturator Oblique Posterior Wall Anterior Column), but not the sacroiliac joint so well; and Iliac oblique, where the pelvis on that side is rotated so that the iliac wing is parallel to the X-ray cassette and the obturator foramen now lies perpendicular to the film, showing the anterior wall and posterior column.

7. **b. FICAT II.**
As long as the femoral head is in the pre-collapse phase and has minimal involvement (<30% ideally) core decompression is likely to be beneficial. Results are still not fully conclusive, but current thinking is that pre-collapse heads may be decompressed successfully, but once the collapse (crescent sign, FICAT III) has appeared, salvage is not possible in this way. Whether or not there should be addition of other products such as bone morphogenic protein or growth factors is still controversial.

8. **c. There is a known organism from preoperative aspirate and the patient has commenced antibiotics.**
Selected patients may undergo single-stage revision, with reported better functional outcome than two-stage revisions. The prerequisites for this are healthy soft tissues, minimal bone loss allowing for cement to be inserted, and a known pathogen with sensitivities. Significant severe bone loss, an unidentified pathogen and the presence of multi-resistant bacteria are contraindications to single-stage revision surgery.

9. **d. Valgus deformity of femoral neck.**
All the above are seen due to remodelling of bone and high vascularity, except a valgus deformity. Typically, varus deformity is seen due to initially osteoporotic change which causes deformity under loading before remodelling into its final shape; this is also responsible for anterolateral diaphyseal bowing. Stress fractures may also be seen on the convex side of the femoral diaphysis. Bone may have lytic lesions or be unusually dense, depending on the activity of the disease process.

10. **e. Pressure from straps of abduction wedge pillow.**
Straps from an abduction wedge pillow may cause local pressure to the common peroneal nerve, rather than the sciatic nerve, at the level of the fibular neck resulting in foot drop. The most commonly injured part of the sciatic nerve is the region which goes on to become the common peroneal nerve. In one study, peroneal palsy was found more commonly after average lengthening of 2.7 cm and sciatic palsy with average lengthening of over 4.4 cm.

11. **d. They are associated with degenerate changes and cysts when due to femoro-acetabular impingement.**
Labral tears are often associated with subtle abnormalities of hip anatomy causing femoro-acetabular impingement (FAI). Painful clicking, snapping and similar symptoms are often due to labral tears in association with FAI. Labral tears may present as groin pain usually in certain positions and repetitive movements such as running.

12. **a. Infection is within 3 weeks of surgery.**
Phillips *et al* found 41% of infections were successfully treated with debridement and antibiotics. Crockarell *et al.* found debridement successful only if performed within 2 weeks of onset of symptoms.

13. b. **Lesser trochanter group**.
There are four main trabecular patterns in the proximal femur. There are two compressive, one tensile, and one greater trochanteric group but none relating specifically to the lesser trochanter.

14. c. **Compression of the lateral cutaneous nerve of thigh**.
The lateral cutaneous nerve of thigh may typically be compressed at several locations, such as the inguinal ligament, by tight belts (e.g. weightlifter's belt), resulting in pain in the anterolateral part of the thigh.

15. a. **Previous formation of heterotopic ossification**.
Although the exact aetiology is poorly understood, if there is a history of heterotopic ossification, then it is very likely to recur at a new site of surgery. Other factors include: ankylosing spondylitis, hypertrophic osteoarthritis, and diffuse idiopathic skeletal hyperostosis, with weaker evidence for extensive soft tissue handling/stripping, or bone debris from reamings. Although patients with head injuries are found to produce extensive calcific deposits a patient would not have elective total hip replacement so soon after significant head injury. Over-expression of bone morphogenetic protein-4 BMP-4) may be implicated in the pathogenesis of heterotopic ossification.

16. d. **Continued as usual**.
Although there is a higher rate of infection in general in rheumatoid patients, continuing their methotrexate at the normal dose has not been shown to affect their risk of infection. Grennan *et al* found that methotrexate made no difference to early infection following elective orthopaedic surgery when two groups were compared, one which continued and a group that didn't; other drugs such as penicillamine, indomethacin, ciclosporin, hydroxychloroquine, chloroquine and prednisolone did increase the early infection risk post-operatively. Conversely, discontinuing their methotrexate may result in disease flare that impedes their post-operative rehabilitation.

17. d. **Hip aspiration**.
Although a radio-labelled white cell scan is more likely to be positive in infection rather than inflammation, it cannot be used to definitively differentiate between the two.
A radionuclide bone scan would appear hot in both conditions. A positive hip aspirate would both identify infection, as well as guide antibiotic treatment. Von Rothenburg *et al* found a Tc-99m-labelled scan had sensitivity of 93% but specificity of 65%. Therefore, a positive result (positive predictive value 63%) may not definitely mean an infection, whereas a negative result (negative predictive value 94%) is likely to help rule out infection.

18. a. **It is best with a polished tapered stem**.
Polished tapered stems such as the Exeter stem are best suited to impaction grafting, as subsidence is expected. This is thought to allow subsidence in the cement mantle, and subject the cement to creep, thereby distributing load evenly and encouraging bone to remodel. Although earlier studies have waned against subsidence, Wraighte *et al* showed that there was no link between subsidence (median 2 mm at 1 year; up to total 10 mm in some patients) and 10-year survival.

19. b. Reduce dislocation by a magnitude of 10.
Although there are many studies, most conclude that there is a beneficial effect of repairing the posterior soft tissue structures. A meta-analysis by Kwon *et al* found that the rate of dislocation reduced from 4.46% to 0.49% if repaired.

20. e. Thickness of HA of at least 50 μm.
Although all these factors are important when considering cementless fixation, they are not all relevant to hydroxyapatite-coated stems, and apply also to other stems such as porous-coated and grit-blasted stems. In a canine model, it has been shown that there is greater total bone apposition and bone ingrowth in implants coated with minimum 50 μm hydroxyapatite at the level of the isthmus and the calcar, although there was no difference between having 50 or 100 μm thickness coating on the amount of bony ingrowth.

21. d. Femoral head/neck junction prominence.
The patient is likely to be suffering from cam-type femoro-acetabular impingement, often presenting secondary to DDH, Perthes, or slipped upper femoral epiphysis, with a head/neck junction prominence that may also lead to labral degeneration, cysts and tear. Degenerate changes at the articular surface in mild DDH is rare in a patient of this age, although cysts may be seen at the head/neck junction if there is impingement.

22. e. Remove metalwork, insert cemented stem passing two cortical thicknesses below lowest screw hole.
There is no need to reinforce the femur externally. A well-cemented stem must pass well past the lowest screw hole to reduce the risk of a stress riser. Hip resurfacing in a patient of this age is not recommended.

23. a. Less in ceramic than polyethylene cups.
The Swedish Hip Registry reports that deep infections are slightly lower with ceramic components. The exact mechanism is unclear, but may be due to bacterial adhesion being poorer on the smoother surface of ceramic components.

24. d. If less than 15°, it is one of the indications for pelvic osteotomy.
This is the angle between a vertical line through the centre of the femoral head and a line connecting the centre of the femoral head to the edge of the acetabulum, used in patients over the age of 5, and useful in adults. Greater than 25° is considered normal, and less than 20° is considered a dysplastic acetabulum. Less than 15° is marked dysplasia, and the patient may benefit from osteotomy of the acetabulum.

25. e. Vascularized fibular graft.
As long as there is no collapse of the femoral head, vascularized fibular graft has been shown to be superior to non-vascularized by reducing progression to collapse, as well as having better Harris Hip Scores.

26. c. Lateral cutaneous nerve of thigh.
The ilio-inguinal approach is an exam favourite. It affords exposure to the inner aspect of the pelvis from the sacroiliac joint all the way to pubic symphysis. The lateral cutaneous nerve of thigh often is in the way and must be sacrificed. Although infrequently used by

most surgeons, it would be worth memorizing the concepts of this approach, particularly the structures at risk in the three 'windows': Lateral – between the iliac wing and the iliopsoas muscle; Middle – between the femoral nerve (iliopsoas muscle) and the external iliac vessels; Medial – between the lymphatics and the rectus abdominus at the level of the pubic tubercle.

27. e. Hydrodynamic.
Although the majority of lubrication in total hip replacements is boundary lubrication, hard-on-hard bearing surfaces, such as metal-on-metal, have been found to have hydrodynamic lubrication during the motion phase of the gait cycle, particularly effective when the prosthesis is polar bearing with high conformity.

28. b. Multiple emboli.
Donaldson *et al* have attempted to define this poorly understood phenomenon: "BCIS is characterized by hypoxia, hypotension or both and/or unexpected loss of consciousness occurring around the time of cementation, prosthesis insertion, reduction of the joint or, occasionally, limb tourniquet deflation in a patient undergoing cemented bone surgery." Current thinking on aetiology leans towards multiple embolic showers of fat, marrow, cement particles, air, bone particles and platelet/fibrin aggregate. Previous theories of methylmethacrylate monomers entering the circulation and causing significant vasodilatation have now largely been discounted in favour of the embolic theory.

29. c. Gluteus maximus and adductor magnus.
The sciatic nerve passes through the interval between piriformis and superior gemellus to lie under gluteus maximus, and passes over the gemelli, obturator internus, and quadratus femoris, before passing over the posterior surface of adductor magnus until it divides into its terminal branches. Cross-sectional anatomy of the limbs at different levels is a popular exam question, and it is worth memorizing the major structures in relation to each other.

30. e. Inwardly displaced parasymphyseal fracture >1 cm.
The single biggest predictor of urethral injury is pubic symphysis diastasis, especially of >1 cm, along with medially displaced medial 1/3 fracture. However, inward displacement didn't result in a large number of patients having urethral injury. It would appear that the traction caused to the urethra is more significant than compression.

EMQs

1. 1. **d. Gluteus maximus and gluteus medius**. 2. **i. Rectus abdominis**. 3. **f. Inguinal ligament**.

Although in reality most of us will rarely use the approach to the pelvis, it is an exam favourite. The Kocher–Langenbeck approach is an extension of the posterior approach to the hip but with elevation of gluteus maximus from the femur, and gluteus maximus and medius from the posterior and lateral ilium, taking care with the superior and inferior gluteal neurovascular bundles. The anterior approach to the pubic symphysis utilizes a curved transverse incision above the symphysis and divides both rectus abdominis muscles entirely, but due to a segmental nerve supply they are not denervated. The bladder lies immediately posteriorly to the pubic symphysis, separated by the space of Retzius. The inguinal ligament, if damaged at its attachment at the anterior superior iliac spine (ASIS), may result in an inguinal hernia, so anterior crest harvesting should not be extended so low.

2. 1. **a. 1, 2, 3**. 2. **e. 6, 7**. 3. **g. 3, 4, 5**.

Gruen zones for femoral stem loosening are 1–7, starting laterally at the greater trochanter and working inferiorly and medially to end at the calcar.

Delee and Charnley zones for acetabular cup loosening are 1–3, commencing at the lateral acetabulum and working medially.

3. 1. **g. Chiari**. 2. **h. Shelf**. 3. **a. Ganz**.

It is worth knowing the main pelvic osteotomies in relation to the age they are performed, indication, whether they are reconstructive or salvage, and the basics of which bones are osteotomized. The Chiari and shelf osteotomies are both salvage procedures, relying on the femoral head being contained in a 'pseudo'-acetabulum; whereas the Ganz osteotomy is technically very challenging but can reorientate the acetabulum very well.

4. 1. **b. 25–30°**. 2. **c. 0–5°**. 3. **c. 0–5°**.

The hip should be in a flexed position to aid ground clearance and sitting position; and avoiding abduction, otherwise an abduction lurch will result. The hip should be in neutral or slight external rotation to allow for pelvic translation during gait.

5. 1. **c. Calcar pivot**. 2. **e. Bending cantilever**. 3. **a. Pistoning: stem and cement within bone**.

Five modes of femoral stem loosening and seven zones of loosening have been described. Calcar pivoting of the stem results in the stem toggling more medially from its original position, i.e. zone 4 at tip and zone 5 medially. Cantilever bending demonstrates good distal fix but toggling mediolaterally at the proximal end. With stem and cement moving as one and pistoning in and out of the bone, all seven zones must be loose; this is different to the stem moving within a fixed cement mantle, which may only show zones 1 and 2 loosening with a distal cement fracture and distal migration of the stem as a result.

6. 1. **e. Rectus femoris**. 2. **f. Hamstrings**. 3. **j. Sartorius**.

Avulsion injuries are being diagnosed more frequently, occurring mainly in adolescents. The mainstay of treatment is non-operative. They usually result in a return to full activity, power and range of movement within a matter of weeks. Large fragments which are significantly displaced or have developed into non-union may occasionally need internal fixation.

7. 1. **e. Urgent/semi-elective internal fixation.** 2. **c. Non-weight-bearing for 2 weeks, then gradual increase in weight-bearing.** 3. **c. Non-weight-bearing for 2 weeks, then gradual increase in weight-bearing.**
Fullerton and Snowdy have classified such stress fractures into type A (lateral/superior neck, under tension), requiring screw fixation; type B (medial/inferior neck, under compression), treated with rest followed by protected weight-bearing; and type C (displaced), requiring internal fixation/replacement as appropriate.

8. 1. **d. Labral tear.** 2. **f. Hamstring avulsion.** 3. **c. Iliotibial band syndrome.**
Iliotibial band syndrome may present as severe snapping at the lateral aspect of the hip, patients may describe the hip feeling as if it has dislocated in severe instances; worse in females with prominent trochanters and running on banked surfaces. Hamstring tears/ avulsions are due to sudden contractures, such as sprinting. Labral tears often present in young patients with no trauma; groin clicking is a sensitive symptom, but may also be frequently caused by iliopsoas over the hip joint.

9. 1. **a. Porosity reduction using a vacuum.** 2. **f. Pulsatile lavage.** 3. **d. Finger packing.**
First generation involved finger packing with no canal preparation or pressurization of cement. Second generation techniques introduced pulsed lavage and canal preparation. With third generation techniques the cement is mixed in a vacuum and pressurized upon insertion.

10. 1. **h. Chordoma.** 2. **a. Chondrosarcoma.** 3. **b. Ewing's sarcoma.**
Chordoma is in the spinal column, often sacrococcygeal and manifests as sacral/pelvic/hip pain or even bowel symptoms. Typically, it has physaliferous cells (bubble-like/vacuolated).

Chondrosarcoma is commonly found in the pelvic girdle, and shows a mineralizing pattern due to its cartilage content. Histology often shows large cells with more than one nucleus.

Ewing's sarcoma should be suspected in the patient younger than 30 years old, particularly with histology showing a 'small round cell tumour'.

11. 1. **h. Titanium head.** 2. **b. Cobalt-chrome acetabular shell with ceramic liner.** 3. **c. Polyethylene socket.**
Bearing surface choices are always controversial. Newer ceramic technologies are very hard wearing but do not have enough long-term survival data to make them comparable with the traditional poly/CoCr combination. The Swedish Hip Registry reports the polyethylene cup as having the lowest revision rate of all combinations over 10 years. Cemented polyethylene cups have a 40% lower revision rate over 10 years than uncemented sockets. Metal-on-metal, although usually aimed at the younger market, is also very useful in those at high risk of dislocation, e.g. Parkinson's, due to the large jump distance required to dislocate. Metal-on-metal articulations such as resurfacings are more likely to produce an immune-mediated aseptic lymphocytic vasculitis-associated lesion (ALVAL) response in young women, as well as elevated blood metal ion levels, and are often avoided for this

reason. Ceramic components are very hard wearing but also brittle, making their toughness low in comparison. They have been known to fracture, thereby making revision extremely challenging once there is ceramic debris within the joint. They are also known to cause squeaking noises. Stripe wear is localized wear thought to occur either during microseparation in the gait cycle, during loading when flexed (e.g. rising from a chair or climbing steep stairs) or due to edge loading of the acetabular component. Although a good choice for femoral stems due to its biocompatibility, titanium is not suitable as a bearing surface due to poor wear resistance. Its surface is easily oxidized to produce a very hard surface; however, the underlying titanium is soft and with movement the surface shears off, exposing the underlying surface, which is oxidized again, resulting in a recurring wear pattern.

12. 1. **c. 50–60%.** 2. **d. 40–50%.** 3. **b. 20–30%.**
After 20 years of follow up, although patients will most frequently experience severe back pain, it is knee or contralateral hip pain that is more likely to require intervention (i.e. total knee replacement (TKR) or total hip replacement (THR)).

13. 1. **g. Coagulase-negative staphylococcus.** 2. **c. Methicillin-sensitive *Staphylococcus aureus*.** 3. **e. *Enterococcus*.**
In a study over 15 years, including 10 735 patients, coagulase-negative staphylococcus was found to cause 36%, *Staphylococcus aureus* 25%, and *Enterococcus* 9% of deep joint infections. MRSA and *Pseudomonas* were responsible only for 4% each.

14. 1. **f. Posterior division of obturator nerve.** 2. **a. Gracilis and adductor longus.** 3. **c. Gluteus medius and tensor fascia lata.**
Approaches to the hip are common topics in the exam. Medial and anterolateral approaches are less frequently used by most surgeons, but should be learnt. The medial (Ludloff) approach is between gracilis and adductor longus superficially, and deeper between adductor brevis and adductor magnus. The posterior division of the obturator nerve may be injured as it lies on adductor magnus, which it supplies, along with branches from the tibial part of the sciatic nerve. Adductor brevis is supplied by the obturator nerve. The anterior branch of the obturator nerve supplies gracilis, adductor longus and adductor brevis. The anterolateral approach is between gluteus medius and tensor fascia lata.

15. 1. **c. 50 μm.** 2. **c. 50 μm.** 3. **e. 150 μm.**
The optimal pore size is 50–150 μm; maximum gap between implant and bone is 50 μm; maximum micromotion is 150 μm; optimal porosity is 40–50%; and optimal thickness of hydroxyapatite if applied is 50 μm.

Selected references

Basta MA, Blackmore CC, Wessels H. Predicting urethral injury from pelvic fracture patterns in male patients with blunt trauma. *J Urol* 2007; 177(2): 571–5.

Board TN, Karva A, Board RE *et al.* The prophylaxis and treatment of heterotopic ossification following lower limb arthroplasty. *J Bone Joint Surg Br* 2007; **89** (4): 434–40.

Callaghan JJ, Brand RA, Pedersen DR. Hip arthrodesis: a long-term follow-up. *J Bone Joint Surg Am* 1985; 67(9): 1328–35.

Canale ST, Beaty JH. *Campbell's Operative Orthopaedics*, 11th edn. Philadelphia, Mosby, 2007.

Clohisy JC, Beaule PE, O'Malley A, *et al*. Hip disease in the young adult: current concepts of etiology and surgical treatment. *J Bone Joint Surg Am* 2008; **90**: 2267–81.

Crockarell JR, Hanssen AD, Osmon DR, Morrey BF. Treatment of infection with debridement and retention of the components following hip arthroplasty. *J Bone Joint Surg Am* 1998; **80**(9): 1306–13.

Damany DS, Parker MJ, Chojnowski A. Complications after intracapsular hip fractures in young adults – a meta-analysis of 18 published studies involving 564 fractures. *Injury* 2005; **36**: 131–41.

DeLee JG, Charnley J. Radiological demarcation of cemented sockets in total hip replacement. *Clin Orthop Relat Res* 1976; **121**: 20–32.

Donaldson AJ, Thomson HE, Harper NJ, Kenny NW. Bone cement implantation syndrome. *Br J Anaesth* 2009; **102**(1): 12–22.

Edwards BN, TullosHS, Noble PC. Contributory factors and etiology of sciatic nerve palsy in total hip arthroplasty. *Clin Orthop Relat Res* 1987; **218**: 136–41.

Fullerton LR, Snowdy HA. Femoral neck stress fractures. *Am J Sports Med* 1988; **16**: 365–77.

Garellick G, Kärrholm J, Rogmark C, Herberts P. *Swedish National Hip Arthroplasty Register Annual Report 2008*. https://www.jru.orthop. gu.se (Accessed 18 March 2011).

Grennan DM, Gray J, Loudon J., Fear S. Methotrexate and early postoperative complications in patients with rheumatoid arthritis undergoing elective orthopaedic surgery. *Ann Rheum Dis* 2001; **60**(3): 214–17.

Gruen TA, McNeicc GM, Amstutz H. "Modes of failure" of cemented stem-type femoral components. A radiographic analysis of loosening. *Clin Orthop Relat Res* 1979; **141**: 17–27.

Hooper ACB. The role of the iliopsoas muscle in femoral rotation. *Ir J Med Sci* 1977; **146**(4): 108–12.

Hoppenfeld S, deBoer P, Buckley R. *Surgical Exposures in Orthopaedics: The Anatomic Approach*, 3rd edn. Philadelphia, Lippincott Williams and Wilkins, 2009.

Karabatsos B, Myerthall SL, Fornasier EL, *et al*. Osseointegration of hydroxyapatite porous-coated femoral implants in a canine model. *Clin Orthop Relat Res* 2001; (**392**): 442–9.

Kwon MS, Kuskowski M, Mulhall KJ *et al*. Does surgical approach affect total hip arthroplasty dislocation rates? *Clin Orthop Relat Res* 2006; **447**: 34–8.

Lieberman JR. Core decompression for osteonecrosis of the hip. *Clin Orthop Relat Res* 2004; **418**: 29–33.

Macfarlane RJ, Haddad FS. The diagnosis and management of femoro-acetabular impingement. *Ann R Coll Surg Engl*. 2010; **92**(5): 363–7.

Manley MT, Sutton K. Bearings of the future for total hip arthroplasty. *J Arthroplasty* 2008; **23**(7 Suppl): 47–50.

Miller MD. *Review of Orthopaedics*, 5th edn. Philadelphia, Elsevier, 2008.

Mulliken BD. Osteonecrosis of the femoral head: current concepts and controversies. *Iowa Orthop J* 1993; **13**: 160–6.

Oussedik SIS, Dodd MB, Haddad FS. Outcomes of revision total hip replacement for infection after grading according to a standard protocol. *J Bone Joint Surg Br* 2010; **92**(9): 1222–6.

Overgaard S, Lind M, Glerup H *et al*. Porous-coated versus grit-blasted surface texture of hydroxyapatite-coated implants during controlled micromotion: mechanical and histomorphometric results. *J Arthroplasty* 1998; **13**(4): 449–58.

Parker MJ, Livingstone V, Clifton R, McKee A. Closed suction surgical wound drainage after orthopaedic surgery. *Cochrane Database Syst Rev* 2007 Jul 18;(3): CD001825.

Phillips JE, Crane TP, Noy M *et al*. The incidence of deep prosthetic infections in a specialist orthopaedic hospital. *J Bone Joint Surg Br* 2006; **88**(7): 943–8.

Plakseychuk AY, Kim S-Y, Park B-C *et al*. Vascularized compared with nonvascularized fibular grafting for the treatment of osteonecrosis of the femoral head. *J Bone Joint Surg Am* 2003; **85**(4): 589–96.

Toms AD, Davidson D, Masri BA, Duncan CP. The management of peri-prosthetic infection in total joint arthroplasty. *J Bone Joint Surg Br* 2006; **88**(2): 149–55.

Upadhyay A, Jain P, Mishra P *et al.* Delayed internal fixation of fractures of the neck of the femur in young adults. A prospective, randomised study comparing closed and open reduction. *J Bone Joint Surg Br* 2004; 86: 1035–40.

von Rothenburg T, Schoellhammer M, Schaffstein J, Koester O, Schmid G. Imaging of infected total arthroplasty with Tc-99m-labeled antigranulocyte antibody Fab'fragments. *Clin Nucl Med* 2004; 29(9): 548–51.

Willert HG, Buchhorn GH, Fayyazi A *et al.* Metal-on-metal bearings and hypersensitivity in patients with artificial hip joints – a clinical and histomorphological study. *J Bone Joint Surg Am* 2005; 87(1): 28–36.

Wraighte PJ, Howard PW. Femoral impaction bone allografting with an Exeter cemented collarless, polished, tapered stem in revision hip replacement: a mean follow-up of 10.5 years. *J Bone Joint Surg Br* 2008; 90(8): 1000–4.

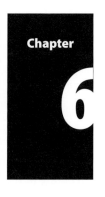

Chapter

6

Knee: Questions

Kesavan Sri-Ram and Howard Ware

MCQs

1. **After cementing in a total knee replacement for a valgus knee, you find that it remains tight laterally in extension. The next most appropriate step is to?**
   a. Carry out a medial release.
   b. Carry out a medial release and increase the size of the polyethylene insert.
   c. Release the iliotibial band.
   d. Release popliteus.
   e. Decrease the size of the polyethylene insert.

2. **Which of the following statements regarding anterior cruciate ligament (ACL) grafts is false?**
   a. The maximum load to failure of a patellar tendon graft is approximately 2600 newtons.
   b. The use of an autologous hamstring graft results in a 50% loss of hamstring strength.
   c. The maximum load to failure of a quadruple hamstring graft is approximately 4500 newtons.
   d. Allograft processing does not always alter the mechanical properties of the graft.
   e. The maximum load to failure of the native ACL is approximately 2100 newtons.

3. **Which of the following is considered to be the primary stabilizer of knee to external rotation?**
   a. Anterior cruciate ligament (ACL).
   b. Posterior cruciate ligament (PCL).
   c. Lateral collateral ligament (LCL).
   d. Medial collateral ligament (MCL).
   e. Patellar tendon.

4. **A 34-year-old man presents with a 3 month history of knee pain, with an inability to squat. The most likely diagnosis is?**
   a. Primary osteoarthritis.
   b. Osteochondral defect.
   c. Loose body.
   d. Posterior horn meniscal tear.
   e. Pigmented villonodular synovitis.

Postgraduate Orthopaedics, ed. Kesavan Sri-Ram. Published by Cambridge University Press.
© Cambridge University Press 2012.

5. **During trialling of a total knee replacement, the knee is tight in extension but correct in flexion. The appropriate step is to?**
   a. Decrease the size of the polyethylene insert.
   b. Resect more distal femur.
   c. Decrease the size of the femoral component.
   d. Resect more proximal tibia.
   e. Resurface the patella to balance the difference.

6. **Which of the following mechanisms best describes the common cause of failure of the polyethylene in a total knee replacement?**
   a. Adhesive wear.
   b. Two-body abrasive wear.
   c. Fatigue wear.
   d. Third-body abrasive wear.
   e. Corrosive wear.

7. **Which of the following is incorrect regarding the native anterior cruciate ligament (ACL)?**
   a. It has an anteromedial bundle which is tight in flexion.
   b. Its length typically ranges from 25 to 41 mm.
   c. Its primary role is proprioceptive.
   d. It has a posterolateral bundle which is tight in extension.
   e. It is supplied by the middle genicular artery.

8. **Which of the following is false regarding the normal anatomy of the knee?**
   a. The patellofemoral ligament is part of layer 2 of the lateral structures of the knee.
   b. The meniscofemoral ligament of Humphrey lies anterior to the ligament of Wrisberg.
   c. The posteromedial bundle of the posterior cruciate ligament is tight in extension.
   d. The superficial medial collateral ligament is part of layer 1 of the medial structures of the knee.
   e. The peripheral portion of the menisci is supplied by the medial and lateral genicular arteries.

9. **Which of the following should be avoided during total knee arthroplasty to avoid lateral patellar subluxation?**
   a. Internal rotation of the tibial component.
   b. External rotation of the femoral component.
   c. Lateral placement of the tibial component.
   d. Lateral placement of the femoral component.
   e. Medial placement of the patellar component.

10. **Which of the following would not be advisable in the treatment of a 45-year-old man with isolated medial compartment osteoarthritis of the knee?**
    a. Non-steroidal anti-inflammatory drugs.
    b. Medial unicompartmental knee replacement.
    c. Autologous chondrocyte implantation.

   d. Opening wedge high tibial osteotomy.
   e. Closing wedge high tibial osteotomy.

11. **A 72-year-old who underwent a total knee replacement 6 weeks ago, presents with increasing knee pain and swelling, with raised inflammatory markers. An aspiration of the joint cultures coagulase-negative staphylococcus. The next most appropriate step in management is?**
   a. Single-stage revision plus intravenous antibiotics.
   b. Two-stage revision, with cement spacer plus intravenous antibiotics.
   c. Intravenous antibiotics.
   d. Open washout/debridement, polyethylene exchange and intravenous antibiotics.
   e. Arthroscopic washout/debridement and intravenous antibiotics.

12. **Regarding total knee replacement, which of the following is incorrect?**
   a. The joint line can be safely lowered 4 mm without an adverse effect on motion and joint instability.
   b. The minimum recommended thickness of an ultra-high-molecular-weight polyethylene insert is 6–8 mm.
   c. A deficient extensor mechanism is a relative contraindication to a total knee replacement.
   d. There is a poorer implant survivorship in patients with rheumatoid arthritis.
   e. Following previous patellectomy, a posterior cruciate ligament-substituting implant is preferred.

13. **The following situations preclude the use of a high tibial osteotomy for the treatment of medial compartment osteoarthritis, except?**
   a. Lateral tibial subluxation.
   b. Lateral compartment osteoarthritis.
   c. Previous subtotal lateral meniscectomy.
   d. Deficient anterior cruciate ligament.
   e. Inflammatory arthropathy.

14. **A 71-year-old patient presents with increasing knee pain 6 weeks after having a total knee replacement. Which of the following would be most reliable in the diagnosis of infection?**
   a. Erythrocyte sedimentation rate.
   b. C-reactive protein.
   c. Microscopy and culture of joint aspirate.
   d. Triple phase isotope bone scan.
   e. Magnetic resonance imaging.

15. **The following are all considered predisposing factors for patellofemoral disorders, except?**
   a. Femoral anteversion.
   b. Lateral patella tilt.
   c. Patella baja.
   d. Reduced trochlea sulcus.
   e. Lateral tibial tuberosity.

16. **Which of the following statements regarding anterior cruciate ligament (ACL) reconstruction is true?**
    a. The femoral tunnel should be in the 1 o'clock position in the right knee.
    b. On the lateral radiograph, the femoral tunnel should be on the anterior half of Blumensaat's line.
    c. On the femoral side, interference screw fixation has been shown to be superior to suspensory type fixation.
    d. During hamstring harvesting, the connection between the semitendinosus and the medial gastrocnemius must be divided.
    e. Hamstring and patellar tendon grafts have an equal tensile strength.

17. **Which of the following is not true of the menisci?**
    a. The lateral meniscus is more mobile than the medial meniscus.
    b. A discoid meniscus is more common in the lateral meniscus.
    c. The collagen content is predominantly type 1.
    d. Their primary role is to provide anteroposterior stability to the knee.
    e. In the developing fetus, the menisci appear by day 45.

18. **An 81-year-old lady is reviewed 6 months after a total knee replacement. Her only complaint is some numbness on the outer aspect of her midline scar. The most likely cause of this is?**
    a. Injury to the femoral nerve from the tourniquet.
    b. Division of the lateral femoral cutaneous nerve.
    c. Injury to the anterior femoral cutaneous nerve from the tourniquet.
    d. Division of the infrapatellar branch of the saphenous nerve.
    e. Injury to the lateral femoral cutaneous nerve from the tourniquet.

19. **A 62-year-old man presents with a painful snapping sensation when extending his knee, 6 months after a posterior stabilized total knee replacement. The most appropriate treatment is?**
    a. Bracing.
    b. Topical anti-inflammatory gels.
    c. Revision of patellar component.
    d. Arthroscopic or open debridement.
    e. Revision of femoral component.

20. **Which of the following is not true of unicompartmental knee replacements?**
    a. Inflammatory arthropathy is a contraindication to unicompartmental knee replacement.
    b. Unicompartmental knee replacements have not been shown to produce better subjective results than total knee replacements.
    c. Patients over 80 years should not have a unicompartmental knee replacement.
    d. A varus deformity of 10° is not a contraindication to unicompartmental knee replacement.
    e. In an anterior cruciate ligament deficient knee, it is reasonable to simultaneously reconstruct the ligament and perform a unicompartmental knee replacement.

21. **Which of the following statements is true regarding mobile-bearing total knee replacements in comparison to fixed-bearing total knee replacements?**
    a. There is a reduction in the amount of volumetric wear.
    b. They result in a better post-operative range of motion.
    c. They result in better post-operative patient-reported outcome scores.
    d. They do not have a better survivorship.
    e. They should only be used in patients under 70 years of age.

22. **A 58-year-old man is listed for a total knee replacement. He underwent a closing wedge high tibial osteotomy 10 years prior. The most likely problem one would encounter during the total knee replacement is?**
    a. Difficult surgical exposure.
    b. Lateral ligament laxity.
    c. Difficult tibial stem placement.
    d. Non-union of the osteotomy.
    e. Patella baja.

23. **Which of the following is true regarding meniscal repair?**
    a. Simultaneous reconstruction of a deficient anterior cruciate ligament has no influence on the success of meniscal repair.
    b. Capsule exposure for an inside-out lateral meniscal repair is performed through the iliotibial band and biceps tendon interval, followed by retraction of the lateral head of the gastrocnemius anteriorly.
    c. Degenerative meniscal tears are a relative contraindication to repair.
    d. Saphenous nerve injury is more common with an all-inside technique compared to an inside-out technique for medical meniscus repair.
    e. Capsule exposure for an inside-out lateral meniscal repair is performed through the lateral head of the gastrocnemius and biceps tendon interval, followed by retraction of the biceps tendon anteriorly.

24. **The surgical approach for the posterior cruciate ligament insertion site during an open inlay technique is?**
    a. A posteromedial approach between medial gastrocnemius and semimembranosus.
    b. A posteromedial approach between medial gastrocnemius and semitendinosus.
    c. A posteromedial approach between semimembranosus and semitendinosus.
    d. A posteromedial approach between splitting medial gastrocnemius.
    e. A posteromedial approach between splitting semimembranosus.

25. **Which of the following is true regarding knee injury in sports?**
    a. Neuromuscular training explains the greater incidence of anterior cruciate ligament injuries in men compared to women in similar sports.
    b. A grade 3 posterior cruciate ligament injury requires reconstruction.
    c. Prophylactic knee bracing in contact sports reduces the incidence of anterior cruciate ligament injuries.
    d. An injury with external tibial rotation with the knee at 90° of flexion is likely to injure the posterior cruciate and lateral collateral ligaments.
    e. There is no gender difference in total varus or valgus knee loading during landing from a jump.

26. **The following is not true of osteochondritis dissecans?**
    a. Open growth plates imply a better prognosis.
    b. Partial detachment of the lesion corresponds to grade III in the Guhl classification.
    c. An 18-year-old would be category II according to the Pappas classification.
    d. The condition is more common in males.
    e. The condition is more common on the lateral than medial femoral condyle.

27. **A 22-year-old man has an arthroscopy 1 year after microfracture treatment for a full-thickness chondral defect. The defect has filled and a biopsy is taken. This is most likely to show?**
    a. Hyaline cartilage.
    b. Fibrocartilage.
    c. Cancellous bone.
    d. Cortical bone.
    e. Elatin.

28. **The blood supply to the anterior cruciate ligament is?**
    a. The medial superior genicular artery.
    b. The lateral superior genicular artery.
    c. The middle genicular artery.
    d. The lateral inferior genicular artery.
    e. The medial inferior genicular artery.

29. **Which statement is incorrect regarding tunnel placement during anterior cruciate ligament reconstruction?**
    a. A femoral tunnel place at the roof of the notch would result in decreased rotational stability.
    b. The posterior cruciate ligament can serve as a reference for tibial tunnel positioning.
    c. The posterior border of the anterior horn of the lateral meniscus can serve as a reference for tibial tunnel positioning.
    d. An anteriorly placed femoral tunnel can result in decreased flexion post-operatively.
    e. Tunnel placement is less important when using synthetic grafts.

30. **An active 66-year-old man is reviewed 1 year after a total knee replacement. He complains that it does not feel right and clinical examination identifies an incompetent medial collateral ligament. The most appropriate treatment is?**
    a. Anti-inflammatory gel and tablets.
    b. Hinged knee brace.
    c. Open repair of the medial collateral ligament.
    d. Reconstruction of the medial collateral ligament.
    e. Revision to a constrained knee prosthesis.

EMQs

1. **Special tests during knee examination**
   a. Lachman test
   b. Anterior drawer test
   c. Pivot shift test
   d. Clark's test
   e. J sign
   f. Apprehension test
   g. McMurray's test
   h. Apley's test
   i. Dial test
   j. Quadriceps active test

Which of the options above is best described in each of the following statements? Each option may be used once, more than once or not at all.
   1. This test would be positive in an isolated posterior cruciate ligament injury without injury to the posterolateral corner.
   2. This is the most sensitive test for anterior cruciate ligament deficiency.
   3. This test is reliant on an intact medial complex and an intact iliotibial band.

2. **Knee injuries**
   a. Anterior cruciate ligament tear
   b. Posterior cruciate ligament tear
   c. Medial collateral ligament tear
   d. Lateral collateral ligament tear
   e. Posterolateral corner injury
   f. Bucket handle tear of the medial meniscus
   g. Lateral meniscal tear
   h. Medial patellofemoral ligament tear
   i. Knee dislocation
   j. Proximal tibiofibular dislocation

Which of the options above is best described in each of the following statements? Each option may be used once, more than once or not at all.
   1. A 15-year-old girl presents with a painful swollen knee following a twisting injury playing basketball. A lateral knee radiograph shows an opacity behind the patella and an MRI shows an osteochondral injury to the lateral femoral condyle. What has she most likely injured?
   2. A 23-year-old rugby player presents with a painful knee after a crunching tackle with a heavy opponent. He has increased anterior and posterior laxity and numbness in his foot. The most likely injury is?
   3. A 29-year-old semi-professional netballer presents with a painful knee with reduced range of motion following a twisting injury. She recalls a severe injury 2 years prior when she landed awkwardly after jumping, but did not receive any treatment. The most likely injury is?

3. **Radiological features of the knee**
   a. Patella baja
   b. Segond sign
   c. Pellegrini–Stieda sign
   d. Patella alta
   e. Blumensaat's line
   f. Insall and Salvati method
   g. Blackburne and Peel method
   h. Squared-off lateral femoral condyle
   i. Appears on three sagittal MRI images
   j. Double posterior cruciate ligament (PCL) sign on MRI

Which of the options above is best described in each of the following statements? Each option may be used once, more than once or not at all.
   1. A radiographic feature of a discoid lateral meniscus.
   2. Small radio-opacity adjacent to the medial femoral condyle.
   3. The ratio between the perpendicular distance from the lower articular margin of patella to the tibial plateau and the length of articular surface of patella.

4. **Surgical options**
   a. Arthroscopic debridement
   b. Microfracture
   c. Proximal tibial osteotomy
   d. Distal femoral osteotomy
   e. Patellofemoral replacement
   f. Unicompartmental knee replacement
   g. Total knee replacement
   h. Anterior cruciate ligament (ACL) reconstruction
   i. Posterior cruciate ligament (PCL) reconstruction
   j. Knee fusion
   k. Revision knee replacement
   l. Amputation

Which of the options above is best described in each of the following statements? Each option may be used once, more than once or not at all.
   1. A 51-year-old lady with rheumatoid arthritis presents with medial knee pain, with radiographs showing complete loss of medial joint space. A recent arthroscopy showed no degeneration in the lateral or patellofemoral compartments.
   2. A 35-year-old man, who is a keen badminton player, presents with medial knee pain, with radiographs showing complete loss of medial joint space, but preserved lateral and patellofemoral compartments.
   3. A 34-year-old medical registrar presents with medial knee pain, with normal looking radiographs. A recent arthroscopy showed a 2 × 2 cm full thickness cartilage defect in the medial femoral condyle.

5. **Knee pathology**
   a. Osteochondritis dissecans
   b. Transient osteoporosis

c. Osteoarthritis
d. Rheumatoid arthritis
e. Psoriatic arthritis
f. Osteonecrosis
g. Medial meniscal tear
h. Lateral meniscal tear
i. Pigmented villonodular synovitis
j. Synovial chondromatosis
k. Synovial sarcoma
l. Parosteal osteosarcoma

Which of the options above is best described in each of the following statements? Each option may be used once, more than once or not at all.
1. A 49-year-old lady presents with a 1 month history of severe medial knee pain, with no history of trauma. Radiographs do not show any adverse features.
2. A 30-year-old lady presents with a 3 month history of knee pain, with no history of trauma. Radiographs show an ossified mass arising from the posterior distal femur.
3. A 32-year-old lady presents with a 6 month history of knee pain, associated with stiffness and recurrent haemorrhagic effusions. Radiographs show cystic erosion with sclerotic margins on both sides of the joint.

6. Fractures around the knee
a. Schatzker type I
b. Schatzker type II
c. Schatzker type III
d. Schatzker type IV
e. Schatzker type V
f. Schatzker type VI
g. Meyers and McKeever type I
h. Meyers and McKeever type II
i. Meyers and McKeever type III
j. Supracondylar
k. Intercondylar

Which of the options above is best described in each of the following statements? Each option may be used once, more than once or not at all.
1. An isolated fracture of the medial tibial plateau.
2. A displaced intercondylar eminence with intact posterior hinge.
3. Generally accepted to be the worst tibial plateau fracture with respect to prognosis.

7. Anatomy of the knee
a. Medial collateral ligament
b. Lateral collateral ligament
c. Anterior cruciate ligament
d. Posterior cruciate ligament
e. Medial meniscus
f. Lateral meniscus

  g. Popliteofibular ligament
  h. Popliteal oblique ligament
  i. Iliotibial band
  j. Medial patellofemoral ligament
  k. Arcuate ligament
  l. Patellar tendon
  m. Quadriceps tendon

Which of the options above is best described in each of the following statements? Each option may be used once, more than once or not at all.
  1. This consists of an anterolateral and posteromedial bundle.
  2. This may cause a positive Ober test if pathological.
  3. A 'Y'-shaped condensation of fibres that runs from the fibular head, over the popliteus, to insert on the posterior capsule.

8. **Scoring systems**
  a. Knee Society Score (KSS)
  b. Oxford Knee Score (OKS)
  c. Knee Injury & Osteoarthritis Outcome Score (KOOS)
  d. Western Ontario and McMaster Universities Osteoarthritis Index (WOMAC)
  e. International Knee Documentation Committee Score (IKDC)
  f. Short Form 12 (SF-12)
  g. Short Form 36 (SF-36)
  h. Tegner Activity Level
  i. Tegner and Lysholm Score

Which of the options above is best described in each of the following statements? Each option may be used once, more than once or not at all.
  1. This is a 12-point subjective only score.
  2. This scoring system involves objective assessment.
  3. This system is helpful when assessing return to sport.

9. **Paediatric knee conditions**
  a. Osteochondritis dissecans
  b. Osgood–Schlatter's disease
  c. Sinding-Larsen–Johansson disease
  d. Tibial eminence fracture
  e. Tibial tubercle fracture
  f. Blount's disease

Which of the options above is best described in each of the following statements? Each option may be used once, more than once or not at all.
  1. A 14-year-old boy injures his knee with a forced flexion mechanism and sustains an Ogden type II injury.
  2. A 13-year-old boy presents with knee pain and a radiograph shows osseous fragmentation of the distal patellar pole.
  3. This condition is associated with an increased Drennan angle.

10. **Balancing a total knee replacement**
    a. Upsize femoral component
    b. Downsize femoral component
    c. Upsize tibial component
    d. Downsize tibial component
    e. Upsize polyethylene insert
    f. Downsize polyethylene insert
    g. Resect more distal femur
    h. Resect more proximal tibia
    i. Medial release
    j. Posteromedial release
    k. Lateral capsular release
    l. Iliotibial band release
    m. Popliteus release
    n. Lateral collateral ligament release

Which of the options above is best described in each of the following statements? Each option may be used once, more than once or not at all.
    1. The components are trialled and the knee is coronally balanced, but tight in flexion and extension. The next step would be.
    2. The components are trialled following cuts and partial releases for a valgus knee. The knee is balanced coronally in extension, but appears tight on the lateral side in flexion. The next step would be.
    3. The same case from question 2 is reassessed and is now coronally balanced in flexion, but is tight compared to extension. The next step would be.

11. **Synovial pathology**
    a. Pigmented villonodular synovitis
    b. Synovial chondromatosis
    c. Juvenile rheumatoid arthritis
    d. Haemophilia
    e. Lipoma arborescens
    f. Gout
    g. Pseudogout

Which of the options above is best described in each of the following statements? Each option may be used once, more than once or not at all.
    1. This results in a haemosiderotic synovitis.
    2. This results in a synovium which has a bright yellow, nodular, papillary appearance.
    3. This condition is associated with crystals which under polarized light microscopy have strong negative birefringence.

12. **Clinical findings**
    a. Grade 1
    b. Grade 2
    c. Grade 3

   d. Grade 4

   e. Grade 5

Which of the options above is best described in each of the following statements? Each option may be used once, more than once or not at all.

1. The knee is flexed to 25° and the tibia translated anteriorly. The tibia translates 7 mm.
2. The knee is flexed to 90° and the anterior surface of the tibia is flush with the femoral condyles.
3. A valgus stress is applied to the knee and this causes pain but there is no excessive movement.

13. **The popliteal fossa**
   a. Popliteal artery
   b. Popliteal vein
   c. Semitendinosus
   d. Tibial nerve
   e. Semimembranosus
   f. Common peroneal nerve
   g. Biceps femoris
   h. Popliteal fascia
   i. Medial head of the gastrocnemius
   j. Femoral artery
   k. Lateral head of the gastrocnemius

Which of the options above is best described in each of the following statements? Each option may be used once, more than once or not at all.

1. This forms the superolateral boundary.
2. This forms part of the roof.
3. This neurovascular structure is anteriormost.

14. **Choice of knee replacement design**
   a. Medial unicompartmental
   b. Lateral unicompartmental
   c. Patellofemoral
   d. Total, posterior cruciate retaining
   e. Total, posterior cruciate substituting
   f. Total, constrained non-hinged
   g. Total, constrained hinged

Which of the options above is best described in each of the following statements? Each option may be used once, more than once or not at all.

1. A 69-year-old lady with rheumatoid arthritis and a painful knee, with radiographs showing diminished joint space in both lateral and medial compartments and neutral alignment.
2. A 67-year-old man with a painful knee and tricompartmental osteoarthritis on radiographs. Thirty years ago he sustained a significant sporting injury

when he hyperflexed his knee with his foot plantarflexed, but did not receive any specific treatment.
3. A 61-year-old man with medial knee pain and slight varus deformity. Radiographs show reduced joint space in the medial compartment and a valgus stress radiographs show reduced joint space in the lateral compartment.

15. The patellofemoral joint and extensor mechanism
   a. Patella dislocation
   b. Lateral patella syndrome
   c. Patella instability
   d. Patellofemoral osteoarthritis
   e. Quadriceps rupture
   f. Patellar fracture
   g. Chondromalacia patellae
   h. Patellar tendinosis
   i. Bipartite patella
   j. Patellar tendon rupture
   k. Patellar sleeve fracture
   l. Multipartite patella

Which of the options above is best described in each of the following statements? Each option may be used once, more than once or not at all.
   1. A 33-year-old lady presents with knee pain, particularly when descending stairs. Her radiographs show patellar tilt in a lateral direction.
   2. A 21-year-old physiotherapist presents with a swollen knee following an injury, but does not recall the mechanism. An MRI shows a structure avulsed from the medial epicondyle of the femur.
   3. A 32-year-old radiology registrar presents with knee pain, and is told their condition is better treated non-operatively nowadays.

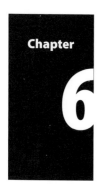

Chapter

6

Knee: Answers

Kesavan Sri-Ram and Howard Ware

MCQs

1. **c. Release the iliotibial band.**
In this situation, it is most appropriate to release the iliotibial band. In general soft tissue releases address coronal imbalance and implant changes address flexion/extension imbalance. For varus deformity/tightness, it is normal to release sequentially as follows: osteophytes, deep medial collateral ligament (MCL) and capsule, semimembranosus, superficial MCL, posterior cructiate ligament (PCL). For valgus deformity/tightness, it is normal to release sequentially as follows: osteophytes, lateral capsule, iliotibial band if tight in extension, popliteus if tight in flexion, lateral collateral ligament (LCL).

2. **b. The use of an autologous hamstring graft results in a 50% loss of hamstring strength.**
In-vitro and cadaveric experiments have identified the approximate ultimate loads of native ACL, patellar tendon grafts and quadruple hamstring grafts to be 2100, 2600 and 4500 newtons respectively. It is important to remember that there are many additional factors which contribute to the final properties of the graft including fixation method and tunnel positioning. Allografts have an important role in both primary and revision ACL reconstruction and their use varies worldwide. Although irradiating allograft can decrease the mechanical properties, fresh frozen grafts preserve their strength. Harvesting autologous hamstrings usually only results in a 10% (approximately) reduction in hamstring strength.

3. **c. Lateral collateral ligament (LCL).**
The knee consists of both primary and secondary stabilizers or restraint to movement, which are as follows:

Movement	Primary stabilizer	Secondary stabilizers
Anterior translation	ACL	iliotibial band (ITB) mid-medial capsule, mid-lateral capsule, MCL, LCL, menisci
Posterior translation	PCL	LCL/posterolateral corner (PLC), MCL
Internal rotation	ACL	popliteal oblique ligaments, posteromedial complex (PMC)

Postgraduate Orthopaedics, ed. Kesavan Sri-Ram. Published by Cambridge University Press.
© Cambridge University Press 2012.

Movement	Primary stabilizer	Secondary stabilizers
External rotation	LCL and popliteofibular ligament	PLC; MCL
Valgus	superficial MCL	PMC, ACL
Varus	PMC, ACL	ACL, PLC

4. **d. Posterior horn meniscal tear.**
The most likely diagnosis here is a tear of the posterior horn of the medial meniscus. The key is the pain when squatting. Primary osteoarthritis is unlikely in a 34-year-old and the other options are possible, but are more likely to present with less specific pain and often swelling.

5. **b. Resect more distal femur.**
It is important to ensure balanced flexion and extension during total knee replacement. As a general rule, if the knee is tight in flexion and extension, the tibia is addressed. If the knee is tight in either flexion or extension, the femur is addressed. There are different methods which may be used including:

Tight in flexion and extension – (i) decrease polyethylene insert size; (ii) resect more proximal tibia

Tight in extension only – (i) resect additional distal femur; (ii) posterior capsular release

Tight in flexion only – (i) downsize the femoral component; (ii) recess and release the posterior cruciate ligament; (iii) resect a posterior slope on the tibia; (iv) release the posterior capsule

6. **c. Fatigue wear.**
Fatigue wear (also referred to as delamination or catastrophic wear) is the usual cause of failure of the polyethylene in total knee replacements. Subsurface failure occurs due to repeated loading, and the surface layer of the polyethylene breaks off. Adhesive wear is due to a junction forming between two surfaces as they come into contact. Two-body abrasive wear relates to wear between two surfaces of different hardness and third-body abrasive wear occurs when extra material appears between two opposing surfaces. Corrosive wear occurs between metals and not polyethylene.

7. **c. Its primary role is proprioceptive.**
Although the ACL has a major role in proprioception, receiving innervation from the tibial nerve, its primary role is as a restraint to anterior tibial displacement. The average length is 38 mm, and it has a small anteromedial and a bulky posterolateral bundle. It arises from a femoral attachment at the posteromedial corner of the medial aspect of the lateral femoral condyle in the intercondylar notch and inserts into a tibial attachment in a fossa in front of and lateral to the anterior tibial spine.

8. **d. The superficial medial collateral ligament is part of layer 1 of the medial structures of the knee.**
The layers of the knee are as follows:

Lateral

> Layer 1 – iliotibial tract, biceps (common peroneal nerve lies between layer 1 and 2)
> Layer 2 – patellar retinaculum, patellofemoral ligament
> Layer 3 superficial – lateral collateral ligament (LCL), fabellofibular ligament (lateral geniculate artery runs between deep and superficial layer)
> Layer 3 deep – arcuate ligament, coronary ligament, popliteus tendon, popliteofibular ligament, capsule

Medial

> Layer 1 – sartorius and fascia (gracilis, semitendinosis, and saphenous nerve run between layer 1 and 2)
> Layer 2 – semimembranosus, superficial medial collateral ligament (MCL), posterior oblique ligament
> Layer 3 – deep MCL, capsule

There are two meniscofemoral ligaments which arise from the posterior horn of the lateral meniscus and insert into the substance of the posterior cruciate ligament; the ligament of Humphrey lies anterior to the ligament of Wrisberg. The posterior cruciate ligament is approximately 38 mm in length and arises from the antero-lateral aspect of the medial femoral condyle in the area of intercondylar notch and inserts into the tibial sulcus, over the back of tibial plateau approximately 1 cm distal to the joint line. It is composed of an anterolateral and posteromedial bundle and is supplied by the middle genicular artery.

9. **a. Internal rotation of the tibial component.**
Patellar maltracking can occur following incorrect component positioning. Internal rotation and medial placement of the femoral component, and lateral placement of the patellar component lead to more lateral alignment of the patella within the trochlear groove. Internal rotation and medial placement of the tibial component lead to a lateralized tibial tubercle, and hence increased Q-angle.

10. **c. Autologous chondrocyte implantation.**
Non-steroidal anti-inflammatory drugs, partial or total knee replacement, and high tibial osteotomy (opening or closing) are acceptable treatment for isolated medial compartment osteoarthritis. Other modalities would include physiotherapy, alternative analgesics, supplements, braces and intra-articular injections. Autologous chondrocyte implantation, whilst shown to be effective for treating isolated chondral defects, is not effective for treating osteoarthritis.

11. **d. Open washout/debridement, polyethylene exchange and intravenous antibiotics.**
This patient presents with an early prosthetic infection. The accepted treatment is an open debridement and intravenous antibiotics. Arthroscopic washout can be effective in some situations, but intravenous antibiotics alone are not likely to be successful. Single or staged revision is acceptable treatment for an infected joint replacement, but would not be used in the first instance, and is reserved for if the initial treatment fails.

12. d. **There is a poorer implant survivorship in patients with rheumatoid arthritis.**

Raising or lowering the joint line during total knee replacement can have an adverse effect on range of motion, patellar function and stability, and can lead to early revision. The accepted safe distance for altering the joint line is 8 mm. The minimum thickness of an ultra-high-molecular-weight polyethylene insert is 6–8 mm; thinner implants are associated with earlier failure due to fatigue wear. Contraindications to total knee replacement include a deficient extensor mechanism, infection, vascular deficiency and neuromuscular abnormalities affecting the muscles around the knee. Patients with rheumatoid arthritis have a lower risk of failure of total knee replacement; other good prognostic variables are age over 60 and use of a condylar prosthesis with a metal-backed tibial component. Following patellectomy, it is thought there are increasing stresses on the posterior cruciate ligament, resulting in deficiency and greater anteroposterior instability if the ligament is not substituted.

13. d. **Deficient anterior cruciate ligament.**

A high tibial, valgus-producing osteotomy, either lateral closing or medial opening, is an effective surgical option for medial compartment osteoarthritis. It suits younger patients with varus alignment, fixed flexion less than 15º and flexion greater than 90º. Contraindications include lateral compartment degeneration, loss of a significant portion of the lateral meniscus, lateral tibial subluxation of greater than 1 cm, medial compartment bone loss, symptomatic patellofemoral degeneration, inflammatory arthritis and poor patient compliance. Anterior cruciate ligament deficiency alone is not a contraindication.

14. c. **Microscopy and culture of joint aspirate.**

The diagnosis of periprosthetic infection soon after surgery is difficult. Both erythrocyte sedimentation rate and C-reactive protein are likely to be elevated due to the post-operative inflammation and a triple phase bone scan would not be able to distinguish between infection and early post-surgical changes. The definitive test in this situation is analysis of a joint aspiration. Radiographs and magnetic resonance imaging are unlikely to be of diagnostic benefit.

15. c. **Patella baja.**

Patellofemoral disorders are extremely common and tend to have a mutlifactorial aetiology. Predisposing factors include the condition femoral anteversion, lateral patella tilt, patella alta (not baja), a reduced trochlea sulcus and a lateral tibial tuberosity. Others include gluteal dysfunction, vastus medialis oblique dysfunction, tight iliotibial band, tight rectus femoris, tight calves/hamstrings, lateral tibial torsion and increased foot pronation.

16. d. **During hamstring harvesting, the connection between the semitendinosus and the medial gastrocnemius must be divided.**

There continues to be debate as to the exact positioning of graft tunnels during ACL reconstruction, but it is generally accepted that the femoral tunnel should be placed posteriorly on the lateral wall of the notch. Therefore, for right knees this is the 10 or 11 o'clock position and for left knees the 1 or 2 o'clock position, and the tunnel should be on the posterior half of Blumensaat's line. There is also debate as to the optimal fixation method, but there is no evidence to support interference being better than suspensory. A number of connections (vinculae) exist with the hamstrings and these must be divided to avoid insufficient harvesting. A fairly predictable vincula exists between semitendinosus and medial gastrocnemius, although anatomical studies have shown that a number of vinculae can be present between both semitendinosus and gracilis and the popliteal fascia, sartorius, gastrocnemius, pretibial and superficial fascia.

17. **d.   Their primary role is to provide anteroposterior stability to the knee**.
The medial meniscus is semicircular in length and about 3 cm long; the lateral meniscus is more circular in shape. The medial meniscus is more fixed than the lateral, which explains the greater incidence of medial meniscal tears compared to lateral. Discoid menisci are more common in the lateral side; the reported incidence is 4–15.5% for lateral versus 0.06–0.3% for medial. The menisci are made up of an extracellular matrix, composed of water and mainly type 1 collagen, as well as glycoproteins, elastin and proteoglycans. The menisci have a number of roles; the principal function is that of load transmission; additional functions are increasing joint conformity, synovial fluid distribution and providing anteroposterior stability.

18. **d.   Division of the infrapatellar branch of the saphenous nerve**.
The anterior cutaneous branches of the femoral nerve consist of the intermediate cutaneous nerve and medial cutaneous nerve. These nerves communicate with the terminal branches of the lateral femoral cutaneous nerve and the infrapatellar branch of the saphenous nerve to form the patellar plexus. The patient's numbness may have been caused by all of the mechanisms described, but with the midline incision for total knee replacement, it is injury to the infrapatellar branch of the saphenous nerve which is the most likely cause.

19. **d.   Arthroscopic or open debridement**.
This patient is describing patellar clunk syndrome. This occurs when a fibrous nodule of tissue forms in the undersurface of the quadriceps tendon just above the patella. It is a problem with posterior stabilized knee replacements but can also occur in cruciate retaining designs. As the knee extends the nodule impinges in box of femoral component and with continued extension it jumps out with an audible or palpable clunk. Non-operative treatment is usually not successful and debridement of the nodule is requited.

20. **c.   Patients over 80 years should not have a unicompartmental knee replacement**.
The contraindications to unicompartmental knee replacement include anterior cruciate deficiency, inflammatory arthropathy, fixed varus deformity and medial or lateral subluxation. Patellofemoral arthritis is not always considered an absolute contraindication. Although often carried out in younger patients, if the indications are correct, a unicompartmental knee replacement can be carried out at any age. There is continued debate about unicompartmental versus total knee replacement and it is the subject of on-going trials. However, there is evidence to support better subjective results in unicompartmental; this may be due to a better 'feel', owing to the fact that both cruciate ligaments are retained. Simultaneous anterior cruciate ligament reconstruction and unicompartmental knee has been described.

21. **d. They do not have a better survivorship.**
A number of theoretical benefits exist with mobile-bearing knee replacements compared to fixed bearing. Although many have demonstrated good results, there is no good evidence to suggest superiority over fixed-bearing implants. This applies to wear, range of motion, objective and subjective outcome scores and implant survival. Although often used in younger patients, there is no contraindication to their use in older patients.

22. **e. Patella baja.**
Total knee replacement after a proximal tibial osteotomy presents a number of technical difficulties. Studies have shown that these knee replacements are more prone to complications such as persisting pain, malalignment and infections. Any number of problems can be encountered during surgery, but the most common is patella baja, seen with both opening and closing wedge osteotomies, although more commonly in the latter. Another important consideration is the change in tibial slope as closing wedge tends to decrease the posterior tibial slope and opening wedge increases it.

23. **c. Degenerative meniscal tears are a relative contraindication to repair.**
Meniscal repairs are increasingly carried out, perhaps due to the introduction of all-inside techniques with various devices. They have not, however, been shown to be more effective than the open techniques. Consistently better results are achieved in younger patients, with relatively fresh peripheral tears, in stable (or stabilized) knees. Tears through degenerate menisci are unlikely to heal. For an inside-out lateral meniscal repair, the capsule is exposed between the iliotibial band and biceps tendon, followed by posterior retraction of the gastrocnemius. Saphenous nerve injury is more common with an inside-out technique compared to an all-inside technique for medical meniscus repair.

24. **a. A posteromedial approach between medial gastrocnemius and semimembranosus.**
The tibial insertion of the posterior cruciate ligament is best exposed through a posteromedial approach between medial gastrocnemius and semimembranosus. The former is retracted laterally and inferiorly, pulling the nerves and vessels out of the way to reach the posteromedial corner of the joint. The posterolateral corner of the joint is exposed between the lateral head of the gastrocnemius and biceps femoris muscle Muscle-splitting approaches are generally not used at the back of the knee.

25. **d. An injury with external tibial rotation with the knee at 90° of flexion is likely to injure the posterior cruciate and lateral collateral ligaments.**
Neuromuscular training indeed explains the gender difference in the incidence of anterior cruciate ligament in similar sports, but it is higher in women. Furthermore, women have a greater total valgus knee loading when landing from a jump. A grade 3 posterior cruciate ligament injury does not necessarily need reconstruction. The majority of grade 1 and 2 injuries can be treated with protected weight bearing and quadriceps rehabilitation. Grade 3 injuries require immobilization in full extension for 2 to 4 weeks to protect the posterior cruciate ligament and the other posterolateral structures presumed to be damaged. Prophylactic knee bracing has not been shown to reduce anterior cruciate ligament injuries in contact sports, but has been shown to reduce medial collateral ligament injuries.

26. e.   **The condition is more common on the lateral than medial femoral condyle.**

Osteochondritis dissecans is a lesion of subchondral bone that results in subchondral delamination and sequestration with or without articular mantle involvement. It is more common in males (5:3), bilateral in 20%, and more common on the medial femoral condyle (4:1). Healing potential is greater in younger patients and open growth plates are considered a good prognostic factor. Pappas classification describes the age at detection: I – below 12 years, II – 12 to 20 years and III – above 20 years. The Guhl classification is based on arthroscopic appearance: I – intact lesion, II – early separation (stable flap), III – partial detachment and IV – complete detachment.

27. b.   **Fibrocartilage.**

Microfracture involves making multiple holes through the subchondral plate at the base of the articular cartilage defect. This allows undifferentiated mesenchymal stem cells to proliferate in the defect, and they subsequently differentiate into fibrocartilage. There is initially a high proportion of type II collagen but this reverts to predominantly type I collagen. The resulting 'cartilage' fill is not as hard wearing as true hyaline cartilage, but the procedure has been shown to produce long-lasting symptomatic relief.

28. c.   **The middle genicular artery.**

The middle genicular artery supplies the anterior and posterior cruciate ligaments and the synovial membrane. The medial superior genicular supplies the vastus medialis, lower femur and the knee joint. The lateral superior genicular supplies the vastus lateralis, lower femur and the knee joint. The medial inferior genicular supplies the upper end of the tibia and the articulation of the knee.

29. e.   **Tunnel placement is less important when using synthetic grafts.**

A femoral tunnel in the roof of the notch (12 o'clock position) would result in a vertical graft. This would restore anteroposterior stability, but would not impact on the rotational stability. Several reference points are described for the tibial tunnel. These include the anterior border of the posterior cruciate ligament (10–11 mm anterior to) and the posterior border of the anterior horn of the lateral meniscus (along a line from this point to the tibial spine). Mal-positioning of the femoral tunnel can limit post-operative range of motion; an anterior tunnel could limit flexion and a posterior tunnel could limit extension. Tunnel placement is probably even more important when using synthetic grafts as these are less forgiving of mal-positioning.

30. e.   **Revision to a constrained knee prosthesis.**

Medial collateral ligament deficiency in a total knee replacement may present with pain, instability or both. A knee brace may provide a temporary solution. Repair or reconstruction of the ligament is unlikely to provide the necessary valgus resistance, and the only sensible option is to revise to a constrained prosthesis. There is some debate as to whether this can be a high posted design (non-linked) or whether it has to be hinged.

EMQs

1. 1. **j. Quadriceps active test**. 2. **a. Lachman test**. 3. **c. Pivot shift test**.
As with most joints, the knee has a number of special examination tests beyond the look, feel and move. Lachman, anterior drawer and pivot shift all assess anterior cruciate deficiency, and the Lachman test is the most sensitive. The pivot shift relies on an intact medial complex and an intact iliotibial band; with the initial valgus and internal rotation force the tibia will be anterolaterally subluxed on the distal femur; with flexion, the iliotibial band goes from an extender to a flexor of the knee and the tibial anterolateral subluxation reduces. Clark's test, apprehension test and J sign refer to the patellofemoral joint. McMurray and Apley's tests are to detect meniscal pathology. The dial test is for posterolateral corner (PLC) injuries; this is carried out prone with the knee at 30° and 90°; in an isolated PLC injury, there is increased external rotation at 30° and to a lesser extent at 90°. In a combined PLC and posterior cruciate ligament (PCL) injury there is further increased external rotation at 90° compared to 30°. The quadriceps active test is positive in PCL injury.

2. 1. **h. Medial patellofemoral ligament tear**. 2. **i. Knee dislocation**. 3. **f. Bucket handle tear of the medial meniscus**.
More often than not the history of the mechanism of injury is sufficient to establish the diagnosis. The first case is a likely patellar dislocation with associated osteochondral fracture of the lateral femoral condyle (often on reduction of the patella), and the additional injury is a tear of the medial patellofemoral ligament. The second case is a likely knee dislocation with rupture of the anterior and posterior cruciate ligaments. In addition the medial collateral ligament or lateral collateral ligament/posterolateral corner would need to be injured as well for the knee to dislocate. Common peroneal nerve (25%) and vascular (30%) injury are commonly associated. The third case describes a previous anterior cruciate ligament injury, with a valgus/external rotation force, which has not been treated. The subsequent loading on the medial meniscus has resulted in a bucket handle tear following a twist, resulting in a locked knee (reduced range of motion). Posterior cruciate ligament tears occur after a direct force to the proximal tibia with flexed knee (e.g. dashboard injury) or in hyperflexion with plantarflexed foot.

3. 1. **h. Squared-off lateral femoral condyle**. 2. **c. Pellegrini–Stieda sign**. 3. **g. Blackburne and Peel method**.
The Segond sign is a small avulsion fracture from the lateral tibia (capsular injury) and indicates an anterior cruciate ligament tear. Pellegrini–Stieda sign is ossification adjacent to the medial femoral condyle and indicates a chronic medial collateral ligament injury. Patella baja refers to a low lying patella and patella alta to a high lying patella. Blumensaat's line is a condensed linear shadow on lateral radiographs of the knee representing the roof of the intercondylar notch; with the knee at 30°, this line should touch the tip of the normal-height patella. The Insall and Salvati method is the ratio of the length of the patella (greatest diagonal length) to the length of the patellar tendon (from its posterior surface from the lower pole of the patella to its insertion on top of the tibial tubercle).The Blackburne and Peel method is the ratio between the perpendicular distance from the lower articular margin of the patella to the tibial plateau and the length of the articular surface of the patella (with the knee in at least 30° of flexion). A squared-off lateral femoral condyle

and menisci appearing on three consecutive sagittal MRI images are both features of a discoid lateral meniscus, although only the former is 'radiographic'. The double PCL sign signifies a displaced bucket handle tear of the meniscus.

4. 1. **g. Total knee replacement**. 2. **c. Proximal tibial osteotomy**. 3. **b. Microfracture**. It is tempting to suggest a unicompartmental knee replacement for the first patient, but her inflammatory arthropathy is a contraindication. The second patient may also benefit from a unicompartmental knee replacement, but his age and expected level of activity would suggest a proximal tibial osteotomy would be more appropriate. Microfracture is proven treatment for localized chondral defects; if necessary this can be combined with ACL reconstruction or proximal tibial osteotomy if the situation requires it.

5. 1. **f. Osteonecrosis**. 2. **l. Parosteal osteosarcoma**. 3. **i. Pigmented villonodular synovitis**. Spontaneous osteonecrosis of the knee (SONK) often occurs in the medial femoral condyle, and presents with acute pain. There may be no precipitating factors, or it may follow trauma (including arthroscopy). Other predisposing factors include corticosteroids, alcohol abuse, sickle cell disease, systemic lupus erythematosus, Caisson disease (barotrauma) and Gaucher's disease. It is best appreciated on MRI. Often the condition is self-limiting, but subchondral microfracture and collapse may necessitate surgical intervention, including arthroplasty.

Parosteal osteosarcoma is a low-grade osteosarcoma, seen more commonly in females, aged 30–40. They occur on the metaphysis of long bones, and the posterior distal femur is the most common site. Radiographs often show a heavily ossified, lobulated mass arising from the cortex. Treatment is with wide excision, with or without endoprosthetic replacement.

Pigmented villonodular synovitis (PVNS) is a monoarticular reactive synovial disease of unknown aetiology, most commonly affecting the knee. Recurrent atraumatic haemarthoses is a characteristic of the condition. MRI provides the best imaging of the nodular synovial proliferation. Treatment involves open or arthroscopic synovectomy, both with high recurrence rates.

6. 1. **d. Schatzker type IV**. 2. **h. Meyers and McKeever type II**. 3. **f. Schatzker type VI**. The Schatzker classification describes tibial plateau fractures as follows:

Type I – lateral split fracture
Type II – split-depressed fracture
Type III – pure depression fracture
Type IV – medial plateau fracture
Type V – bicondylar fracture
Type VI – metaphyseal–diaphyseal disassociation

Like many good classifications, the Schatzker classification system is helpful for assessing the initial injury, planning management and predicting prognosis.

The Meyers and McKeever classification describes intercondylar eminence (tibial spine) fractures as follows:

Type I – Minimal displacement of the avulsed fragment, with bony apposition.
Type II – Displacement of the anterior third or half of the affected bone (with intact posterior hinge), with a beaklike deformity appearing on the lateral radiograph.
Type III – Fragment of bone completely separated from its bone bed in the intercondylar eminence, without bony apposition.

7. 1. **d. Posterior cruciate ligament**. 2. **i. Iliotibial band**. 3. **k. Arcuate ligament**.
The posterior cruciate ligament consists of an anterolateral and posteromedial bundle and the anterior cruciate ligament consists of an anteromedial and posterolateral bundle. The anterior bundles are tight in flexion and the posterior bundles are tight in extension. The Ober test is used to detect iliotibial band syndrome, a condition often seen in runners and cyclists, caused by rubbing between the iliotibial band and the lateral femoral condyle. The test involves laying the patient on their side, and extending the knee while bringing it from abduction to adduction; a positive test is associated with pain, tightness or a click. Treatment involves physiotherapy, local corticosteroid or surgery. The iliotibial band arises from the anterior iliac crest outer lip, anterior border of the ilium and outer surface of the anterior superior iliac spine and inserts proximally into the lateral epicondyle of the femur then passes in its broad expansion between the lateral aspect of the patella and inserts distally on Gerdy's tubercle on the lateral aspect of the tibial tubercle. The arcuate ligament is not a separate ligament, but a 'Y'-shaped condensation of fibres that runs from the fibular head, over the popliteus, to insert on the posterior capsule. The popliteofibular ligament runs from the popliteus tendon to the fibular head. The oblique popliteal ligament is a thickening of the medial capsular ligament attached proximally to the adductor tubercle of the femur and distally to the posteromedial aspect of the tibia and posterior aspect of the capsule.

8. 1. **b. Oxford Knee Score (OKS)**. 2. **a. Knee Society Score (KSS)**. 3. **h. Tegner Activity Level**.
Outcome measures and scoring systems are important in orthopaedics and their use is probably on the rise. Although a detailed knowledge of each score is not required, it is helpful to have some basic principles. Scores can be subjective (patient dependent) or objective (examiner assessed) or mixed. They can be general or joint specific, and they can be general or disease specific. In the list provided, all of the scores are knee specific except the SF12 and SF36 which are general and not disease specific. WOMAC is specific for osteoarthritis (although there is a WOMAC for the hip as well). The OKS is a 12-point score. The KSS is the only system in the list that has objective assessment. The Tegner Activity Level describes activity level with respect to work and sport, and therefore is helpful to assess return to sport.

9. 1. **e. Tibial tubercle fracture**. 2. **c. Sinding-Larsen–Johansson disease**. 3. **f. Blount's disease**.
Sinding-Larsen–Johansson disease is an overuse traction apophysitis caused by repetitive microtrauma at the insertion point of the proximal patellar tendon onto the lower patellar pole. Osgood–Schlatter's disease is an overuse traction apophysitis involving the tibial tubercle. The Ogden classification refers to tibial tubercle avulsion fractures, and is as follows:

Type I – a fracture of the secondary ossification centre near the insertion of the patellar tendon.
Type II – the fracture propagates to proximal to the junction with the primary ossification centre.
Type III – the fracture extends posteriorly to cross the primary ossification centre.

An additional A implies undisplaced and B implies displaced.

The Drennan angle is the metaphyseal–diaphyseal angle and is greater than 16° in Blount's disease. This is a pathological genu varum caused by a dyschondrosis of the medial physis of the proximal tibia.

10. 1. **h. Resect more proximal tibia**. 2. **m. Popliteus release**. 3. **b. Downsize femoral component**.

Strategies for balancing a total knee replacement in the coronal and sagittal planes are discussed in the first part of the chapter. The first case being tight in flexion and extension suggests the tibia should be addressed, i.e. more proximal tibia needs to be resected (or in theory, the polyethylene insert can be downsized). The second case is tight laterally in flexion, and so the popliteus is released. It is then tight in flexion, and balanced in extension, and so the femoral component should be downsized (or the posterior cruciate could be recessed and released).

11. 1. **d. Haemophilia**. 2. **e. Lipoma arborescens**. 3. **f. Gout**.

Sufferers of haemophilia are predisposed to recurrent haemathroses of the knee, and this can result in a haemosiderotic synovitis. Lipoma arborescens is a rare disease of the synovium in which there is fatty infiltration of the subsynovial connective tissue. Macroscopically, the synovium appears bright yellow with a nodular, papillary appearance. It differs from pigmented villonodular synovitis as it does not have the golden-brown colour. Gout is a crystal arthopathy due to monosodium urate crystals, which display strong negative birefringence under polarized light, in contrast to pseudogout, caused by calcium pyrophosphate crystals, which display weakly positive birefringence.

12. 1. **b. Grade 2**. 2. **b. Grade 2**. 3. **a. Grade 1**.

This question is describing three of the special tests on examination, and relies on recalling the grading of each. The first is the Lachman test for the anterior cruciate ligament and is graded:

Grade 0 – no laxity
Grade 1 – less than 0.5 cm of translation
Grade 2 – 0.5–1.0 cm of translation
Grade 3 – 1.0–1.5 cm of translation

The second is the posterior drawer for the posterior cruciate ligament and is graded:

Grade 0 – tibia should lie 1 cm anterior to the femoral condyles
Grade 1 – laxity compared with the other knee, but the tibia remains anterior to the femoral condyles
Grade 2 – the anterior surface of the tibia and femoral condyles are flush
Grade 3 – tibia can be translated posterior to the femoral condyles

The third is the valgus stress test for the medical collateral ligament and is graded:

Grade 1 – pain, but no opening up
Grade 2 – some opening up, but with an end point
Grade 3 – more opening up with no end point

13. 1. **g. Biceps femoris**. 2. **h. Popliteal fascia**. 3. **a. Popliteal artery**.

The popliteal fossa is the space located at the back of the knee joint. The boundaries are semitendinosus and semimembranosus (superomedial), biceps femoris (superolateral), medial head of the gastrocnemius (inferomedial) and lateral head of the gastrocnemius muscle and plantaris (inferolateral). The roof is formed by the skin, superficial fascia and the popliteal fascia. The floor is formed by the popliteal surface of femur, the joint, the oblique popliteal ligament and the fascia covering the popliteus. The fossa contains the popliteal artery (most anterior), the popliteal vein, the tibial and common peroneal nerves and lymph nodes.

14. 1. **e. Total, posterior cruciate substituting**. 2. **e. Total, posterior cruciate substituting**. 3. **d. Total, posterior cruciate retaining**.

Unfortunately, there is controversy as to the choice of implant in many cases. However, traditional teaching suggests that a posterior cruciate substituting design should be used in inflammatory arthritis, post-patellectomy, post posterior cruciate ligament (PCL) rupture and post excessive PCL release during knee balancing. Of course, many surgeons use a posterior cruciate substituting design in all cases. In the third case, it is tempting to consider a medial unicompartmental design, but the valgus radiograph precludes this.

15. 1. **b. Lateral patella syndrome**. 2. **a. Patella dislocation**. 3. **h. Patellar tendinosis**.

A number of predispositions lead to patellofemoral problems and include, passive lateral hypermobility (ligamentous laxity), dysplastic vastus medialis obliquis muscle, lateral displacement of patella, patella alta, lateral femoral condyle hypoplasia and increased Q-angle. This last feature is exacerbated by femoral anteversion, genu valgum, external tibial torsion and pronated feet. In the first case the lateral patellar tilt on radiographs suggest this is lateral patella syndrome. The second case describes an avulsion of the medial patellofemoral ligament in association with a patella dislocation. This ligament arises from the medial epicondyle immediately superior to the attachment of the medial collateral ligament and inserts to the superomedial border of the patella, approximately 1 cm distal to the superior pole. The third case has patellar tendinosis. Traditionally, this was treated surgically with variable results. However, a randomized controlled trial has shown no advantage with surgical treatment compared with eccentric strength training.

Selected references

Ayers DC, Dennis DA, Johanson NA, Pelligrini VD. Common complications of total knee arthroplasty. *J Bone Joint Surg Am* 1997; **79**: 278–311.

Bahr R, Fossan B, Løken S, Engebretsen L. Surgical treatment compared with eccentric training for patellar tendinopathy (Jumper's Knee). A randomized, controlled trial. *J Bone Joint Surg Am* 2006; **88**(8): 1689–98.

Blackburne JS, Peel TE. A new method of measuring patellar height. *J Bone Joint Surg Br* 1977; **59**(2): 241–2.

Canale ST, Beaty JH. *Campbell's Operative Orthopaedics*, 11th edn. Philadelphia, Mosby, 2007.

Hoppenfeld S, deBoer P, Buckley R. *Surgical Exposures in Orthopaedics: The Anatomic Approach*, 3rd edn. Philadelphia, Lippincott Williams and Wilkins, 2009.

Insall J, Salvati E. Patella position in the normal knee joint. *Radiology* 1971; **101**(1): 101–4.

Leone JM, Hanssen AD. Management of infection at the site of a total knee arthroplasty. *J Bone Joint Surg Am* 2005; **87** (10): 2335–48.

Meyers, MH, McKeever FM. Fracture of the intercondylar eminence of the tibia. *J Bone Joint Surg Am* 1959; **41**: 209–22.

Miller MD. *Review of Orthopaedics*, 5th edn. Philadelphia, Elsevier, 2008.

Newman J, Pydisetty RV, Ackroyd C. Unicompartmental or total knee replacement:

the 15-year results of a prospective randomised controlled trial. *J Bone Joint Surg Br* 2009; **91**(1): 52–7.

Noyes FR, Butler DL, Grood ES, Zernicke RF, Hefzy MS. Biomechanical analysis of human ligament grafts used in knee-ligament repairs and reconstructions. *J Bone Joint Surg Am* 1984; **66**(3): 344–52.

O'Connell JX. Pathology of the synovium. *Am J Clin Pathol* 2000; **114**(5): 773–84.

Paletta GA Jr, Laskins RS. Total knee arthroplasty after a previous patellectomy. *J Bone Joint Surg Am* 1995; 77: 1708–12.

Pandit H, Beard DJ, Jenkins C, Kimstra Y, Thomas NP, Dodd CA, Murray DW. Combined anterior cruciate reconstruction and Oxford unicompartmental knee arthroplasty. *J Bone Joint Surg Br* 2006; **88**(7): 887–92.

Rand JA, Ilstrup DM. Survivorship analysis of total knee arthroplasty: cumulative rates of survival of 9200 total knee arthroplasties. *J Bone Joint Surg Am* 1991; **73**: 397–409.

Schatzker J, McBroom R, Bruce D. The tibial plateau fracture. The Toronto experience 1968–1975. *Clin Orthop Relat Res* 1979; (**138**): 94–104.

Smith H, Jan M, Mahomed NN, Davey JR, Gandhi R. Meta-analysis and systematic review of clinical outcomes comparing mobile bearing and fixed bearing total knee arthroplasty. *J Arthroplasty* 2011 (in press)

Windsor RE, Bono JV. Infected total knee replacements. *J Am Acad Orthop Surg* 1994; **2**: 44–53.

Woo SL, Hollis JM, Adams DJ, Lyon RM, Takai S. Tensile properties of the human femur-anterior cruciate ligament-tibia complex. The effects of specimen age and orientation. *Am J Sports Med* 1991; **19**(3): 217–25.

Wright JM, Crockett HC, Slawski DP, Madsen MW, Windsor RE. High tibial osteotomy. *J Am Acad Orthop Surg* 2005; **13**(4): 279–89.

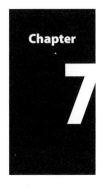

Chapter

Foot and ankle: Questions

Kesavan Sri-Ram and Andrew Robinson

MCQs

1. **Which of the following nerves supply the greatest area of sensibility of the foot?**
   a. Sural.
   b. Saphenous.
   c. Tibial.
   d. Deep peroneal.
   e. Superficial peroneal.

2. **A 32-year-old man sustains a Lisfranc fracture dislocation. Which of the following is the most important factor in predicting a satisfactory outcome?**
   a. Severity of initial injury.
   b. The state of the articular cartilage.
   c. The age of the patient.
   d. The smoking status of the patient.
   e. Whether or not a compensation claim is involved.

3. **Which of the following is not typically associated with a ball and socket ankle joint?**
   a. Absent fibula.
   b. Deficient knee ligaments.
   c. An equinovarus deformity.
   d. Talocalcaneal coalition.
   e. Proximal femoral focal deficiency.

4. **A vertical talus is most commonly associated with which of the following?**
   a. Oligohydramnios.
   b. Arthrogryposis.
   c. Congenital talipes equinovarus.
   d. Tarsal coalition.
   e. Developmental dysplasia of the hip.

5. **A 13-year-old girl who enjoys ballet presents with a painful big toe whilst performing. The likely diagnosis is?**
   a. Hallux valgus.
   b. Hallux rigidus.

Postgraduate Orthopaedics, ed. Kesavan Sri-Ram. Published by Cambridge University Press.
© Cambridge University Press 2012.

   c. Sesamoid fracture.
   d. Turf toe.
   e. Extensor hallucis longus rupture.

6. **Which of the following inserts into the talus?**
   a. Tibialis anterior.
   b. Tibialis posterior.
   c. Extensor digitorum longus.
   d. Extensor digitorum brevis.
   e. None of the above.

7. **Which of the following ossification centres is first to appear?**
   a. Intermediate cuneiform.
   b. Medial cuneiform.
   c. Lateral cuneiform.
   d. Cuboid.
   e. Navicular.

8. **Which of the following has two ossification centres?**
   a. Talus.
   b. Cuboid.
   c. Navicular.
   d. Lateral cuneiform.
   e. Calcaneum.

9. **A 27-year-old banker injures his foot and sustains a displaced divergent Lisfranc fracture-dislocation. The optimal management would consist of?**
   a. Below knee plaster cast.
   b. A bridging external fixator.
   c. Closed or open reduction and K-wire stabilization.
   d. Closed or open reduction and screw stabilization.
   e. Closed or open reduction and combined screw and K-wire stabilization.

10. **The Lisfranc ligament's attachments are?**
   a. Intermediate cuneiform to base of second metatarsal on plantar surface.
   b. Medial cuneiform to base of second metatarsal on plantar surface.
   c. Medial cuneiform to base of second metatarsal on dorsal surface.
   d. Intermediate cuneiform to base of first metatarsal on dorsal surface.
   e. Medial cuneiform to base of first metatarsal on plantar surface.

11. **A 22-year-old radiographer injures his ankle after a twisting injury whilst snowboarding. He has been diagnosed with a ligament injury, but 8 weeks after injury has continued lateral pain. The most likely diagnosis is?**
   a. Lateral malleolus fracture.
   b. Fracture of the lateral process of the talus.
   c. Fracture of the body of the talus.
   d. Fracture of the neck of the talus.
   e. Peroneus longus rupture.

12. **Which of the following is the most common primary soft tissue malignancy of the foot?**
    a. Malignant melanoma.
    b. Osteosarcoma.
    c. Squamous cell carcinoma.
    d. Synovial cell sarcoma.
    e. Chondrosarcoma.

13. **Which of the following is not supplied by branches of the tibial nerve?**
    a. First lumbrical.
    b. Third lumbrical.
    c. Extensor digitorum brevis.
    d. Abductor hallucis.
    e. Abductor digiti minimi.

14. **During ankle arthroscopy, which nerve is most likely to be injured with the anterolateral portal?**
    a. Intermediate dorsal cutaneous branch of the superficial peroneal nerve.
    b. Saphenous nerve.
    c. Sural nerve.
    d. Deep peroneal nerve.
    e. Medial dorsal cutaneous branch of the superficial peroneal nerve.

15. **Which of the following statements regarding hallux valgus is incorrect?**
    a. A long first ray predisposes to hallux valgus.
    b. The intermetatarsal angle is normally less than 10°.
    c. In a hallux valgus deformity, a normal distal metatarsal articular angle implies an incongruent joint.
    d. A post-operative cock-up toe deformity is due to damage to the extensor hallucis longus.
    e. The dorsomedial cutaneous branch of the superficial peroneal nerve is at risk during surgery.

16. **An 11-year-old boy presents with a wound on the sole of his foot after stepping on a nail in the garden, whilst wearing training-shoes. Which organism would you be most concerned about?**
    a. *Staphylococcus aureus*.
    b. *Staphylococcus epidermidis*.
    c. *Pseudomonas aeruginosa*.
    d. *Pasteurella multocida*.
    e. Beta-haemolytic streptococci.

17. **Which of the following is true of talar neck fractures?**
    a. If a displaced talar neck fracture is reduced and stably fixed, the chance of subtalar arthritis is 25%.
    b. A type III fracture is associated with tibiotalar dislocation.
    c. A Hawkins sign seen on a radiograph 6 weeks post-injury is a poor prognostic sign.
    d. Type I and II fractures may be treated non-operatively.
    e. A varus malunion causes decreased eversion.

18. **Which of the following ligaments attaches to the sustentaculum tali?**
    a. Cervical.
    b. Bifurcate.
    c. Long plantar.
    d. Short plantar.
    e. Spring.

19. **A 29-year-old male badminton player presents after an ankle injury. He describes feeling as if someone kicked him in the back of the ankle. What is the most important benefit of surgical treatment for this patient?**
    a. Quicker return to sport.
    b. Decreased risk of chronic pain.
    c. Decreased risk of re-injury.
    d. Decreased risk of nerve damage.
    e. Decreased immobilization time.

20. **Which of the following best describes a low transverse fibular fracture and vertical medial malleolar fracture?**
    a. Supination-external rotation.
    b. Supination-adduction.
    c. Pronation-external rotation.
    d. Pronation-abduction.
    e. Pronation-dorsiflexion.

21. **Which of the following is not a typical deformity seen in congenital talipes equinovarus?**
    a. Forefoot adduction.
    b. Forefoot pronation.
    c. Midfoot cavus.
    d. Hindfoot varus.
    e. Hindfoot equinus.

22. **A 23-year-old presents with on-going pain and stiffness four months after a severe ankle sprain. A radiograph shows a Berndt and Harty type IV lesion of the lateral talar dome. The optimal management would be?**
    a. Below knee weight-bearing plaster cast or protective boot.
    b. Below knee non-weight-bearing plaster cast or protective boot.
    c. Arthroscopy, excision and microfracture.
    d. Arthroscopy and internal fixation.
    e. Open reduction and internal fixation.

23. **Which of the following is not true of tibialis posterior tendon dysfunction?**
    a. It is associated with the 'too many toes' sign.
    b. It has been classified by Johnson and Strom.
    c. Operative treatment may involve a medial displacement calcaneal osteotomy.
    d. A University of Colorado Biomechanics Laboratory orthosis is often effective treatment.
    e. An acute tendon rupture does not result in an immediate flatfoot.

24. **Which structure is most likely to prevent reduction of an ankle dislocation after a supination injury?**
    a. Anterior talofibular ligament.
    b. Calcaneofibular ligament.
    c. Posterior talofibular ligament.
    d. Peroneus brevis tendon.
    e. Tibialis posterior tendon.

25. **Which of the following is incorrect regarding Achilles tendon surgery?**
    a. A posteromedial incision is often used to prevent sural nerve injury.
    b. An end-to-end repair is possible if the smallest gap achievable is 3 cm.
    c. The optimum post-repair position of the foot is 20° plantarflexion.
    d. A V-Y advancement of the gastrocnemius would be required if the smallest gap achievable is 6 cm.
    e. Percutaneous surgery increases the risk of sural nerve injury.

26. **Which of the following is the optimal position for ankle arthrodesis?**
    a. 5° varus, 10° external rotation, 0° flexion, 5 mm anterior talar translation.
    b. 5° valgus, 10° external rotation, 10° dorsiflexion, 5 mm anterior talar translation.
    c. 5° valgus, 10° external rotation, 0° flexion, 5 mm posterior talar translation.
    d. 5° varus, 10° internal rotation, 0° flexion, 5 mm posterior talar translation.
    e. 5° valgus, 10° external rotation, 10° dorsiflexion, 5 mm posterior talar translation.

27. **Which of the following is not a compartment of the foot?**
    a. Calcaneal.
    b. Interosseus.
    c. Abductor.
    d. Medial.
    e. Lateral.

28. **Which of the following is true of calcaneal fractures?**
    a. They are typically associated with an increased Bohler's angle.
    b. They are extra-articular in the majority of cases.
    c. The Sanders classification is based upon the number and location of articular fragments on sagittal CT scan.
    d. The wound complication rate is 5% following open reduction and internal fixation.
    e. Bilateral fractures occur in 5–10% of cases.

29. **A 12-year-old boy presents with a painful flatfoot. Lateral radiographs show an 'anteater' sign. The most likely diagnosis is?**
    a. Plantar fasciitis.
    b. Accessory navicular.
    c. Tibialis posterior rupture.
    d. Talocalcaneal coalition.
    e. Calcaneonavicular coalition.

30. **Which of the following best describes a toe deformity where there is hyperextension at the metatarsophalangeal joint, flexion at the proximal interphalangeal joint and flexion at the distal interphalangeal joint?**
    a. Claw toe.
    b. Hammer toe.
    c. Mallet toe.
    d. Curly toe
    e. Bunionette.

EMQs

1. **Plantar layers of the foot**
   a. First layer
   b. Between first and second
   c. Second layer
   d. Between second and third
   e. Third layer
   f. Between third and fourth
   g. Fourth layer

Which of the options above is best described in each of the following statements?
Each option may be used once, more than once or not at all.
   1. A muscle, which is not supplied by the tibial nerve or its branches.
   2. A group of muscles supplied by both the medial and lateral plantar nerves.
   3. The muscles related to the knot of Henry.

2. **Angles on radiographs**
   a. Hallux valgus angle
   b. Intermetatarsal angle
   c. Distal metatarsal articular angle
   d. Kite's angle
   e. Bohler's angle
   f. Angle of Gissane
   g. Calcaneal pitch angle
   h. Fowler–Philip's angle
   i. Hibbs' angle
   j. Meary's angle

Which of the options above is best described in each of the following statements?
Each option may be used once, more than once or not at all.
   1. On a lateral radiograph, this is the angle between the downward slope of the posterior facet of the calcaneum and the upward slope of the anterior process of the calcaneum.
   2. On a standing lateral radiograph, this is the angle between the plantar cortex of the calcaneum and a line parallel to the floor.
   3. On an anteroposterior radiograph of the foot, the angle between a line bisecting the head and neck of the talus and a line running parallel with the lateral surface of the calcaneum.

3. **Nerves in the foot**
   a. Common peroneal nerve
   b. Deep peroneal nerve
   c. Superficial peroneal nerve
   d. Tibial nerve
   e. Lateral plantar nerve
   f. Medial plantar nerve
   g. Medial calcaneal nerve

h. Saphenous nerve
i. Sural nerve

Which of the options above is best described in each of the following statements? Each option may be used once, more than once or not at all.

1. This nerve travels between flexor digitorum brevis and abductor hallucis.
2. This nerve would need to be intact for a successful tendon transfer for a foot drop.
3. Entrapment of this nerve's first branch is a cause of medial heel pain.

4. **Painful foot in a child**
    a. Freiberg's disease
    b. Kohler's disease
    c. Sever's disease
    d. Iselin's disease
    e. Os trigonum
    f. Os peroneum
    g. Os vesalianum
    h. Accessory navicular
    i. Tarsal coalition
    j. Turf toe

Which of the options above is best described in each of the following statements? Each option may be used once, more than once or not at all.

1. A 13-year-old boy presents with lateral foot pain, and is tender over the fifth metatarsal. Radiographs show a traction epiphysitis.
2. A 5-year-old boy presents with a limp and painful foot. Radiographs show sclerosis, fragmentation, and flattening of the navicular.
3. A 16-year-old girl complains of pain at the back of her foot, especially when she goes in to *en pointe* position during ballet.

5. **Surgical procedures in the foot and ankle**
    a. Modified Broström
    b. Scarf
    c. Jones
    d. Girdlestone–Taylor
    e. Watson-Jones
    f. Lapidus
    g. Evans
    h. Chrisman–Snook
    i. Modified McBride
    j. Keller
    k. Mitchell's
    l. Akin

Which of the options above is best described in each of the following statements? Each option may be used once, more than once or not at all.

1. A 28-year-old lady presents with a bunion. Clinically she has a hypermobile first ray, and radiographs reveal an intermetatarsal angle of 22°.

2. A 31-year-old man presents with ankle instability and varus stress radiographs of the ankle show a varus tilt.
3. A 54-year-old lady presents with a second toe deformity. There is excessive flexion at the proximal interphalangeal joint, but this corrects passively.

6. **Examination of the foot and ankle**
   a. Coleman block test
   b. Silfverskiold test
   c. Grind test
   d. Simmonds' test
   e. Thompson test
   f. Anterior drawer
   g. Mulder's click
   h. Single leg heel raise
   i. Talar tilt
   j. Homan's sign
   k. The squeeze test

Which of the options above is best described in each of the following statements? Each option may be used once, more than once or not at all.
   1. This tests the integrity of the anterior talofibular ligament.
   2. This tests the integrity of the ankle syndesmosis.
   3. This test is useful for assessing an equinus deformity.

7. **Percentages in foot and ankle**
   a. 5%
   b. 10%
   c. 25%
   d. 40%
   e. 50%
   f. 60%
   g. 75%
   h. 85%
   i. 90%
   j. 100%

Which of the options above is best described in each of the following statements? Each option may be used once, more than once or not at all.
   1. The reduction in tibiotalar contact area following an ankle injury and 1 mm shift of the talus.
   2. The likelihood of avascular necrosis after a talar neck fracture with associated subtalar, tibiotalar and talonavicular dislocation.
   3. The likelihood of osteomyelitis in a diabetic with a foot ulcer with exposed bone.

8. **The diabetic foot**
   a. Eichenholtz stage 0
   b. Eichenholtz stage 1
   c. Eichenholtz stage 2

  d. Eichenholtz stage 3
  e. Wagner and Meggitt grade 0
  f. Wagner and Meggitt grade 1
  g. Wagner and Meggitt grade 2
  h. Wagner and Meggitt grade 3
  i. Wagner and Meggitt grade 4
  j. Wagner and Meggitt grade 5

Which of the options above is best described in each of the following statements? Each option may be used once, more than once or not at all.

  1. A 53-year-old diabetic lady presents with an ulcer on the sole of her foot, with a tendon visible.
  2. A 66-year-old diabetic man presents with an abnormally shaped foot and his radiographs suggest absorption of osseous debris and fusion of larger fragments.
  3. A 55-year-old diabetic man has a very prominent first metatarsal head on the sole of his foot, with haemosiderin deposits in the skin.

9. Treatment of injuries
  a. A non-weight-bearing, below knee cast
  b. A weight-bearing, below knee cast
  c. A non-weight-bearing, above knee cast
  d. A weight-bearing, above knee cast
  e. A removable protective boot
  f. Reduction and percutaneous wires
  g. Open reduction and internal fixation
  h. Open repair
  i. Primary arthrodesis
  j. Amputation

Which of the options above is best described in each of the following statements? Each option may be used once, more than once or not at all.

  1. A 24-year-old professional skier twists her ankle and presents with lateral pain and weakness in eversion. An MRI shows a dislocated peroneus brevis tendon.
  2. A 31-year-old lawyer twists his ankle and presents with a painful swollen ankle. He is very tender over the lateral malleolus and deltoid ligament. A radiograph shows a fracture of the lateral malleolus at the level of the syndesmosis, with a small amount of talar shift.
  3. A 41-year-old car salesman falls from a ladder and injures his ankle. Radiographs show a medial subtalar dislocation. It is reduced under sedation in casualty.

10. Painful foot in an adult
  a. Hallux rigidus
  b. Mallet toe
  c. Tibialis posterior tendon insufficiency
  d. Achilles tendonosis

   e. Plantar fasciitis
   f. Flexor hallucis longus impingement
   g. Gout
   h. Morton's neuroma
   i. Midfoot osteoarthritis
   j. Haglund's deformity
   k. Ankle osteoarthritis
   l. Talar osteochondral lesion

Which of the options above is best described in each of the following statements?
Each option may be used once, more than once or not at all.
  1. A 23-year-old professional dancer complains of pain in her foot, particularly when *en pointe*.
  2. A 21-year-old complains of pain at the back of his foot after exercise and has a bump on the back of his heel.
  3. A 41-year-old man complains of heel pain, which is worse in the morning, better during the day and bad again in the evenings.

11. **Insertion of tendons**
   a. Lateral malleolus
   b. Medial malleolus
   c. Talus
   d. Calcaneum
   e. Cuboid
   f. Navicular
   g. Lateral cuneiform
   h. Intermediate cuneiform
   i. First metatarsal
   j. Fifth metatarsal

Which of the options above is best described in each of the following statements?
Each option may be used once, more than once or not at all.
  1. The peroneus brevis.
  2. The peroneus longus.
  3. The tibialis anterior.

12. **Surgical approaches**
   a. Anterior approach to the tibia
   b. Anterolateral approach to the tibia
   c. Posterolateral approach to the tibia
   d. Lateral approach to the fibula
   e. Lateral approach to the lateral malleolus
   f. Anteromedial approach to the medial malleolus
   g. Posteromedial approach to the medial malleolus
   h. Anterior approach to the ankle
   i. Posterolateral approach to the ankle
   j. Posterior approach to the ankle
   k. Lateral approach to the hindfoot (Ollier's)

Which of the options above is best described in each of the following statements? Each option may be used once, more than once or not at all.
1. This approach uses the interval between peroneus tertius and peroneus brevis.
2. This approach uses the interval between flexor hallucis longus and the peroneal muscles.
3. This approach uses the interval between extensor hallucis longus and extensor digitorum longus.

13. **Radiological classification of hallux valgus**
   a. 3°
   b. 5°
   c. 8°
   d. 11°
   e. 18°
   f. 21°
   g. 24°
   h. 30°
   i. 34°
   j. 39°
   k. 45°

Which of the options above is best described in each of the following statements? Each option may be used once, more than once or not at all.
1. The intermetatarsal angle in a mild deformity.
2. The hallux valgus angle in a mild deformity.
3. The intermetatarsal angle in a moderate deformity.

14. **Ligaments around the ankle**
   a. Anterior-inferior tibiofibular ligament
   b. Anterior talofibular ligament
   c. Posterior-inferior tibiofibular ligament
   d. Posterior talofibular ligament
   e. Transverse tibiofibular ligament
   f. Calcaneo-fibular ligament
   g. Lateral talocalcaneal ligament
   h. Deltoid ligament
   i. Interosseous ligament

Which of the options above is best described in each of the following statements? Each option may be used once, more than once or not at all.
1. This ligament is most commonly injured in an ankle sprain.
2. At the ankle, this ligament is the primary restraint to inversion in plantarflexion.
3. This ligament provides the greatest resistance to movement at the inferior tibiofibular joint.

15. **Inflammatory conditions**
   a. Rheumatoid arthritis
   b. Gout

c. Ankylosing spondylitis
d. Psoriatic arthropathy
e. Systemic lupus erythematosus
f. Diffuse idiopathic skeletal hyperostosis
g. Reiter's syndrome
h. Lyme disease
i. Pseudogout

Which of the options above is best described in each of the following statements? Each option may be used once, more than once or not at all.
1. A 38-year-old man presents with a painful fourth toe, which, on examination, is red and cylindrically enlarged.
2. A 26-year-old man presents with heel pain after running, and on direct questioning describes back stiffness as well.
3. A 31-year-old man with a painful heel is referred by a urologist.

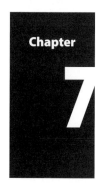

Foot and ankle: Answers

Kesavan Sri-Ram and Andrew Robinson

MCQs

1. c. Tibial.
The tibial nerve supplies nearly all of the sole of the foot through its branches: medial calcaneal, medial plantar and lateral plantar nerves. The sural nerve supplies the lateral border of the foot and the saphenous nerve supplies the medial border and medial aspect of the dorsum. The deep peroneal nerve supplies the dorsal aspect of the first web space and the superficial peroneal nerve supplies the rest of the dorsum.

2. e. Whether or not a compensation claim is involved.
Lisfranc injuries refer to injuries of the tarsometatarsal joint and can range from a mild sprain to dislocation, with or without fracture. The commonest mechanism of injury is indirect, with axial loading or twisting of a hyperplantarflexed foot. The outcome following such an injury is affected by many variables and certainly the severity of the injury, the patient's age and sex, and the adequacy of the reduction are important prognostic factors. Calder and colleagues showed that the presence of a compensation claim is associated with a particularly poor prognosis. Nevertheless it should be borne in mind that Myerson *et al.* found that the quality of the initial reduction was the most important factor in producing an excellent or good clinical result. Furthermore, they concluded that there is no place for conservative management of displaced fractures or fracture-dislocations of the Lisfranc joint.

3. c. An equinovarus deformity.
A ball and socket ankle joint may be congenital or acquired. The latter is very unusual, for example following a subtalar fusion at a very young age. Thus a ball and socket ankle joint is most often associated with congenital abnormality. Causes include fibular hypoplasia, leg length discrepancy, anteromedial tibial bowing, absent lateral rays of the foot, tarsal coalition, deficient knee ligaments and femoral deficiency. The ball and socket ankle tends to be associated with a valgus, as opposed to a varus foot.

4. b. Arthrogryposis.
Congenital vertical talus is a rare disorder of the foot, presenting as a rigid, rocker-bottomed flatfoot. This foot shape is as a consequence of an irreducible dorsal dislocation of the navicular on the talus. The hindfoot is in fixed equinovalgus, the midfoot is dorsiflexed and the forefoot is abducted and dorsiflexed. Approximately 60% of babies suffering from this condition are found to have arthrogryposis or a myelomeningocele.

Postgraduate Orthopaedics, ed. Kesavan Sri-Ram. Published by Cambridge University Press.
© Cambridge University Press 2012.

5. d. Turf toe.
A turf toe refers to a hyperdorsiflexion injury of the first metatarsophalangeal joint, although it is often used to refer to any sprain of that join. In ballet dancers, it is seen as an overuse injury. The plantar plate and sesamoid complex is injured. There may be associated phalangeal stress fractures, sesamoid fractures, and metatarsophalangeal joint degeneration may develop as a late sequelae.

6. e. None of the above.
The talus is made up of a head, neck, body and posterior process. It articulates with the tibia and fibula in the ankle, and the navicular and calcaneum in the foot. It has many ligamentous attachments but no muscle attachments. There is a groove posteriorly in which the flexor hallucis longus tendon runs. It is important to be aware of the blood supply of the talus; the primary source is the artery of the tarsal canal (derived from the posterior tibial artery); additional supply is from the superior neck vessels (derived from the anterior tibial artery) and the artery of the sinus tarsi (derived form the dorsalis pedis).

7. d. Cuboid.
The calcaneum (anterior), talus and cuboid ossification centres are usually present at birth. The lateral cuneiform appears during the first year, the medial cuneiform appears during the second year, the intermediate cuneiform and navicular appear during the third year and the posterior calcaneal centre appears during the eighth year.

8. e. Calcaneum.
Each of the tarsal bones has one ossification centre except the calcaneum, which has an anterior and posterior centre.

9. e. Closed or open reduction and combined screw and K-wire stabilization.
The tarsometatarsal joint is best thought of in three columns: a medial column (first tarsometatarsal joint), a middle column (second and third tarsometatarsal joints) and a lateral column (fourth and fifth tarsometatarsal joints). Any dislocation or subluxation needs reduction. A cast or external fixator does not hold the reduction adequately. Although there are many ways to stabilize the fracture-dislocation after reduction, it is generally accepted that the medial and middle columns should be treated with permanent fixation (for example screws) and the lateral column should have temporary fixation (for example K-wires removed after 6–12 weeks). This is due to the relatively greater mobility of the lateral column.

10. b. Medial cuneiform to base of second metatarsal on plantar surface.
The Lisfranc ligament is a strong oblique ligament, which arises from the plantar-lateral aspect of the medial cuneiform, passes in front of the intercuneiform ligament, and inserts into the plantar-medial aspect of the second metatarsal. In about 20% of patients, there are two separate bands of the ligament (dorsal and plantar).

11. b. Fracture of the lateral process of the talus.
This mechanism of injury is typical for a lateral process of the talus fracture. These injuries are common in snowboarders. The mechanism involves dorsiflexion, axial loading, inversion and external rotation. They are often missed and may require MRI, CT or bone scanning

to make the diagnosis. Undisplaced fractures can be treated in a cast. Displaced fractures (>2 mm) should be reduced and fixed, or excised if they are too small for fixation.

12. d.   Synovial cell sarcoma.

Although primary cutaneous melanoma is the most common malignant tumour of any type in the foot (acral lentiginous melanoma), the most common primary soft tissue malignant tumour in the foot is synovial sarcoma. They make up approximately 8–10% of all sarcomas and most commonly affect adults in the third to fifth decades of life. They are often seen as soft tissue swelling with calcification on plain radiographs. The characteristic histological feature is a biphasic pattern with an epithelial component and a spindle cell component. Other common tumours or tumour-like conditions in the foot include enchondroma, osteoid osteoma, fibrous dysplasia, adamantinoma, osteochondroma, ganglion, clear cell sarcoma and fibromatosis.

13. c.   Extensor digitorum brevis.

The tibial nerve divides into the medial calcaneal (sensory), medial plantar and lateral plantar nerves after it passes behind the medial malleolus. The medial plantar nerve supplies the flexor digitorum brevis, first lumbrical, flexor hallucis brevis and abductor hallucis. The lateral plantar nerve supplies the abductor digiti minimi, flexor digiti minimi brevis, interossei, second to fourth lumbricals, adductor hallucis and flexor digitorum accessorius. The extensor digitorum brevis is supplied by the deep peroneal nerve.

14. a.   Intermediate dorsal cutaneous branch of the superficial peroneal nerve.

The two most common portals used in ankle arthroscopy are the anterolateral and anteromedial. The anterolateral portal is established medial to the lateral malleolus and lateral to the peroneus tertius, and risks injury to the intermediate dorsal cutaneous branch of the superficial peroneal nerve. The anteromedial portal is made lateral to the medial malleolus and medial to tibialis anterior, and risks injury to the saphenous nerve and vein. The anterocentral portal, medial to extensor digitorum longus and lateral to extensor hallucis longus, risks damaging the deep peroneal nerve and anterior tibial artery.

15. d.   A post-operative cock-up toe deformity is due to damage to the extensor hallucis longus.

A post-operative cock-up toe deformity is as a result of inadvertent damage to flexor hallucis longus. The intermetatarsal angle, between the long axes of the first and second metatarsals, is normally less than 10°, and is increased in hallux valgus and used to determine the severity of the deformity. The distal metatarsal articular angle (DMAA) is between the long axis of the first metatarsal and a line through the base of the distal articular cap. It is usually less than 15°. In a hallux valgus deformity with a normal DMAA, the joint is incongruent, whereas in a deformity with an increase in DMAA, the joint is congruent. The dorsomedial cutaneous branch of the superficial peroneal nerve is at risk during surgery, and damage to it can result in a painful neuroma; it is best to undertake a true medial incision, rather than a dorsomedial incision.

16. c.   *Pseudomonas aeruginosa.*

Although the most common organisms responsible for infections after penetrating wounds are *Staphylococcus aureus*, beta-haemolytic streptococci and various anaerobic bacteria,

Pseudomonas aeruginosa is usually responsible for infection when the injury is the result of object penetration through shoes and socks. Such infection may present a few days or weeks after the injury, with pain and swelling. It requires surgical debridement and intravenous antibiotics. *Pasteurella multocida* is seen after dog or cat bites, and puncture wounds from claws.

17. e.   A varus malunion causes decreased eversion.
Talar neck fractures are the commonest fracture of the talus, and follow forced dorsiflexion with axial load. They present a difficult problem, mainly due to the high complication rate, particularly osteonecrosis and post-traumatic osteoarthritis. The Hawkins classification is used for these fractures:

  I – undisplaced
  II – associated subtalar dislocation
  III – associated subtalar and tibiotalar dislocation
  IV(added by Canale) – associated subtalar, tibiotalar and talonavicular dislocation

Type I injuries can be treated non-operatively, but the others need reduction and fixation. Hawkins sign refers to a subchondral lucency see on an anteroposterior radiograph at 6 to 8 weeks, and represents resorption, implying good vascularity, and hence is a good prognostic sign. A varus malunion occurs in one-third of cases and results in decreased eversion.

18. e.   Spring.
The intertarsal ligaments in the foot are important for stability. The cervical is also termed the interosseous talocalcaneal. The bifurcate is composed of two ligaments, which are also termed calcaneocuboid and calcaneonavicular. The long plantar is also termed calcaneocuboid-metatarsal: it arises from the calcaneum and inserts into the cuboid and all five metatarsals. The short plantar is the plantar calcaneocuboid. The spring ligament is the plantar calcaneonavicular and arises from the sustentaculum tali.

19. c.   Decreased risk of re-injury.
This patient has an Achilles tendon rupture. Operative and non-operative management are both acceptable options, but the principal advantage of the former is a decreased risk of re-rupture. This benefit has to be balanced against the complications of surgery, which include wound breakdown, infection and nerve injury. Some of these risks may be reduced by performing surgery percutaneously. Pain and speed of recovery are not necessarily improved by surgery. Surgery may allow a shorter immobilization time, but this is not the principal benefit.

20. b.   Supination-adduction.
An understanding of the Lauge-Hansen classification of ankle fractures is needed to answer this question. The first word in each type refers to the foot's position at the time of injury and the second word refers to the direction of the deforming force. A supination-adduction gives rise to the injury described.

21. b.   Forefoot pronation.
Congenital talipes equinovarus (clubfoot) is a deformity of the foot with an incidence of 1 in 250–1000. It is more common in males and is often bilateral. There may be associated

musculoskeletal anomalies. A number of deformities are seen: forefoot adduction (tibialis posterior), forefoot supination (tibialis anterior), midfoot cavus (intrinsics, flexor hallucis longus, flexor digitorum longus), hindfoot varus (Achilles tendon, tibialis posterior) and hindfoot equinus (Achilles tendon). Dr Ponseti has revolutionized the treatment of clubfoot from a surgical (posteromedial release) to a non-surgical one (serial casting).

22. c. **Arthroscopy, excision and microfracture**.
The Berndt and Harty classification refers to osteochondral lesions of the talus. It is a radiographic classification:

> I – compression of the subchondral bone
> II – a partially detached osteochondral fracture
> III – completely detached, non-displaced fragment
> IV – a detached and displaced osteochondral fragment

Osteochondral lesions of the talar dome are commonly anterolateral or posteromedial; they are often traumatic in origin, particularly the anterolateral lesions, but may also have an osteonecrosis/atraumatic aetiology. Type IV lesions are best treated by excision and microfracture, with good results in up to 86% of patients. Microfracture is usually undertaken arthroscopically. If simple debridement and microfracture is ineffective in reducing symptoms, chondral or osteochondral grafting is considered. Ankle arthrodesis or arthroplasty is the definitive treatment.

23. d. **A University of Colorado Biomechanics Laboratory orthosis is often effective treatment**.
Tibialis posterior tendon dysfunction is very common and often misdiagnosed as a 'sprain' or 'arthritis'. Johnson and Strom described three stages and Myerson added a fourth:

> I – tenosynovitis, normal tendon length, no deformity
> II – tendon lengthening, flexible planovalgus deformity
> III – rigid planovalgus deformity
> IV – valgus ankle tilt

The 'too many toes' sign refers to the number of toes seen from behind; normally up to three, but with a planovalgus deformity, more may be seen. Treatment is always non-operative in the first instance, and can include a University of California (not Colorado) Biomechanics Laboratory heel cup orthosis. Surgery may include tendon debridement, tendon reconstruction, medial displacement calcaneal osteotomy, lateral column lengthening and triple or pantalar arthrodesis. If the tendon is acutely ruptured, which is rare, the flatfoot develops over time as the static stabilizers fail. Normally the tibialis posterior stabilizes the midtarsal joint, if it is absent or defunctioned the midtarsal joint is overloaded and the static supporters (spring ligament, talonavicular capsule, plantar fascia) fail. The arch eventually collapses and a flatfoot ensues.

24. d. **Peroneus brevis tendon**.
This is an uncommon scenario, but is most likely to be caused by interposition of the peroneus brevis tendon. The ankle ligaments do not usually prevent reduction. The tibialis posterior tendon is unlikely to be the cause, although it has been reported as a cause of an irreducible ankle dislocation.

25. **d. A V-Y advancement of the gastrocnemius would be required if the gap is 6 cm**.
Repair of an Achilles tendon is usually undertaken with the patient prone, and an
incision just medial to midline to avoid sural nerve injury. Immobilizing the foot in
20° plantarflexion allows maximum skin perfusion over the tendon, by decreasing skin
tension, and protects the tendon repair. A direct repair is usually possible if the gap is less
than 3 cm. A V-Y advancement of the gastrocnemius can be considered if the gap is between
3 and 5 cm, and if greater than 5 cm, a flexor hallucis longus transfer must be considered.

26. **c. 5° valgus, 10° external rotation, 0° flexion, 5 mm posterior talar translation**.
It is extremely important to fuse the ankle in the correct position. The position affects knee
function and the ability to walk on uneven ground. The ideal position of arthrodesis is
neutral flexion, 0–5° valgus of hindfoot valgus, 5–10° of external rotation, and slight
posterior displacement of the talus under the tibia (5 mm). Posterior displacement
normalizes the gait pattern and decreases the stress on the knee.

27. **c. Abductor**.
There is no abductor compartment in the foot. Traditionally, nine compartments are
described. The names and muscular contents are:

Calcaneal – quadratus plantae
Interosseus (×4) – interossei
Adductor – adductor hallucis
Medial – flexor hallucis brevis, abductor hallucis
Lateral – abductor digiti minimi, flexor digiti minimi
Superficial – flexor digitorum brevis, lumbricals, flexor digitorum longus

28. **e. Bilateral fractures occur in 5–10% of cases**.
Calcaneal fractures occur after an axial load and are bilateral in 5–10% of cases. They are
associated with a spinal injury in about 10%. The majority (75%) are intra-articular, and result
in a decreased Bohler's angle (line drawn by connecting the anterior process, highest point
on posterior articular surface and superior tuberosity on the lateral radiograph). The Sanders
classification is based upon the number and location of articular fragments on the coronal CT
scan, with four types, based on the number of fragments of the posterior facet, with
displacement of 2 mm considered significant. The wound complication rate is reported to
be up to 30%.

29. **e. Calcaneonavicular coalition**.
A painful flatfoot in a child is likely to be secondary to a tarsal coalition. The two commonest
tarsal coalitions are talocalcaneal and calcaneonavicular. The anteater sign is visualized on a
lateral radiograph of the foot, and is caused by the elongated anterior process of the calcaneum.
It is associated with a calcaneonavicular coalition. The coalition may be fibrous, cartilaginous
or osseous. Observation, orthoses or plaster immobilization are the initial management
modalities. If non-operative treatment fails, surgical excision and soft tissue interposition
is an option, although arthrodesis may be required if degenerative changes are present.

30. **a. Claw toe**.
These features describe a claw toe deformity. A hammer toe is only flexed at the proximal
interphalangeal joint and a mallet toe is only flexed at the distal interphalangeal joint.
A bunionette is characterized by a prominence of the fifth metatarsal head.

EMQs

1. 1. **g. Fourth layer**. 2. **c. Second layer**. 3. **c. Second layer**.
The layers of the foot are as follows:

Dorsal layer – extensor digitorum brevis

First plantar layer – abductor hallucis, flexor digitorum brevis, abductor digiti minimi

Second plantar layer – quadratus plantae, lumbricals, flexor digitorum longus, flexor hallucis longus

Third plantar layer – flexor hallucis brevis, adductor hallucis, flexor digit minimi brevis

Fourth plantar layer – interossei, peroneus longus, tibialis posterior

The peroneus longus is in layer 4 and supplied by the superficial peroneal nerve. The lumbricals, in layer 2, are supplied by both the medial (first) and lateral (second to fourth) plantar nerves. The flexor hallucis longus and flexor digitorum longus cross at the knot of Henry.

2. 1. **f. Angle of Gissane**. 2. **g. Calcaneal pitch angle**. 3. **d. Kite's angle**.
The hallux valgus angle (anteroposterior (AP)) is the angle between the longitudinal axes of the first metatarsal and proximal phalanx, and is normally less than 15°. It is increased in hallux valgus.

The intermetatarsal angle (AP) is the angle between the longitudinal axes of the first and second metatarsal, and is normally less than 10°. It is increased in hallux valgus.

The distal metatarsal articular angle (AP) is the angle between the distal articular surface of the first metatarsal head and the long axis of the first metatarsal. It is normally less than 10°, and is increased in congruent hallux valgus. It is also known as the proximal articular set angle.

Kite's talocalcaneal angle (AP) is the angle between a line bisecting the head and neck of the talus and a line running parallel with the lateral surface of the calcaneum, it is normally less than 20–40°. It is decreased in clubfoot.

Bohler's angle is the angle between a line between the anterior process of the calcaneum and the highest point of the posterior articular surface, and a line connecting the highest point on the posterior articular surface and superior tuberosity on the lateral radiograph. It is normally 25–40°, and is decreased in intra-articular calcaneal fractures.

The angle of Gissane is the angle between the downward slope of the posterior facet of the calcaneum and the upward slope of the anterior calcaneal process. It is normally 120–145° if increased in joint depression fractures of the calcaneum.

The calcaneal pitch angle is the angle between the plantar cortex of the calcaneum and a line parallel to the floor. It is normally 10–30° if decreased in pes planus and increased in pes cavus.

Fowler–Philip's angle is the angle between a line tangential to the anterior tubercle and the plantar tuberosity of the calcaneum and a line tangential to the posterior prominence at the insertion of the Achilles tendon. It is normally 45–70°, and increased with a Haglund's deformity.

Hibbs' angle is the angle between the axes of the calcaneum and the first metatarsal, on a lateral radiograph, and is normally less than 130°. It is decreased in pes cavus and increased in pes planus.

Meary's angle is the angle measured on a lateral weight-bearing radiograph, between the long axes of the talus and first metatarsal, and is normally 0°. It flattens with pes planus and steepens with pes cavus.

3. 1. **f. Medial plantar nerve**. 2. **d. Tibial nerve**. 3. **e. Lateral plantar nerve**.
The medial plantar nerve travels between flexor digitorum brevis and abductor hallucis, whereas the lateral plantar nerve remains deep to both. The tibial nerve, which supplies the tibialis posterior, would need to be intact. A tibialis posterior tendon transfer is a common transfer for a foot drop. Entrapment of the first branch of the lateral plantar nerve (Baxter's nerve), which supplies abductor digiti quinti muscle, can cause plantar, medial heel pain. The compression usually occurs between the abductor hallucis muscle and the quadratus plantae muscle.

4. 1. **d. Iselin's disease**. 2. **b. Kohler's disease**. 3. **e. Os trigonum**.
Iselin's disease is a traction epiphysitis of the fifth metatarsal and may present with lateral foot pain. Os vesalianum may also present with lateral foot pain, but the os is a sesamoid in the peroneus brevis, and appears as an ossicle adjacent to the fifth metatarsal. Sclerosis, fragmentation, and flattening of the navicular are typical of Kohler's disease, an avascular condition of unknown aetiology. Kohler's disease affects boys more than girls, typically between 2 and 7 years of age. The os trigonum is an accessory bone found just posterior to the talus. It is an accessory ossification centre of the posterior process of the talus, and may present with pain, especially when the ankle is plantarflexed, for example in the *en pointe* position. Freiberg's disease is an avascular condition of the second metatarsal head. Sever's disease is a calcaneal apophysitis and causes heel pain. An os peroneum is located in the peroneus longus, as it passes under the lateral aspect of the cuboid.

5. 1. **f. Lapidus**. 2. **a. Modified Broström**. 3. **d. Girdlestone–Taylor**.
The Lapidus procedure is a corrective first tarsometatarsal joint fusion, for the treatment of hallux valgus in association with a hypermobile first ray. The modified Broström procedure is a direct repair of the deficient anterior talofibular and calcaneofibular ligaments. It is usually reinforced by advancing the extensor retinaculum over the repair (the Gould modification). This is an anatomical procedure, and does not compromise the peroneal tendons. It is often the first line for treating patients with ankle instability. Other reconstructive options exist but require a tenodesis using the peroneus brevis; of these the Chrisman–Snook is preferred as it is an anatomical reconstruction. The Watson-Jones and Evans procedure are largely historical. The Girdlestone–Taylor procedure involves a flexor digitorum longus (FDL) to extensor hood transfer, and is used to treat flexible claw and hammer toes. The transferred FDL plantarflexes the proximal phalanx at the metatarsophalangeal joint and extends it at the proximal interphalangeal joint.

6. 1. **f. Anterior drawer**. 2. **k. The squeeze test**. 3. **b. Silfverskiold test**.
In the anterior drawer test the examiner subluxes the ankle forwards with the knee flexed at 60° and the ankle plantarflexed at 10°. It is a test for the anterior talofibular ligament. The talar tilt test assesses the calcaneofibular ligament. The syndesmosis is assessed by the squeeze test, which is performed by compressing the fibula and the tibia together at the mid-tibia. The Silfverskiold test is undertaken with an equinus deformity to assess if the contracture is as a result of gastrocnemius tightness. If the gastrocnemius is relaxed, by flexing the knee, the equinus deformity is correctable with a gastrocnemius contracture, whereas with Achilles tendon tightness the equinus persists with the knee flexed. The Coleman block test is used in the assessment of a cavus foot. With the patient standing a block is placed under the lateral column of the foot. This leaves the medial column and

the first ray unsupported. This eliminates the effect of the first ray in driving hindfoot varus. Thus, if when viewed from behind the heel moves into neutral or valgus, and the subtalar joint is flexible, the plantarflexed first ray is the driver of the heel varus. The grind test assesses metatarsophalangeal degeneration; the joint is moved whilst being longitudinally compressed. Simmonds' and Thompson's tests are used in Achilles ruptures. Mulder's click test is undertaken with the forefoot being squeezed from side to side, and the interspace is balloted; a Morton's neuroma is felt to click. The single leg heel raise assesses the useful tibialis posterior, which initiates this movement.

7. 1. **d. 40%**. 2. **j. 100%**. 3. **h. 85%**.
A 1 mm talar shift will reduce the ankle contact area by 42%. The ankle is a highly conforming joint, which under normal loads maximizes contact areas; this explains the rarity of primary ankle osteoarthritis. This reduction in contact area with only a small amount of talar shift emphasizes the importance of accurate fracture reduction in the treatment of ankle fractures.

Following a talar neck fracture, the approximate risk of avascular necrosis, according to the Hawkins classification is:

Type I (undisplaced) – 0–13%
Type II (subtalar dislocation) – 20–50%
Type III (subtalar and tibiotalar dislocation) – 20–100%
Type IV (subtalar, tibiotalar, and talonavicular dislocation) – 100%

In a diabetic foot ulcer, visible or palpable bone implies an 85% chance of osteomyelitis.

8. 1. **g. Wagner and Meggitt grade 2**. 2. **c. Eichenholtz stage 2**. 3. **e. Wagner and Meggitt grade 0**.
The Eichenholtz classification describes the evolution of a Charcot neuroarthropathy of the foot and has three stages:

Stage 1 – destruction/developmental (acute) – diffuse swelling, joint laxity, subluxation, frank dislocation, fine periarticular fragmentation, debris formation
Stage 2 – coalescence (quiescent) – absorption of osseous debris, fusion of larger fragments, sclerosis
Stage 3 – consolidation (resolution) – osseous remodelling

Eichenholtz "stage 0" has come into use to describe a swollen, hot, and painful foot in which plain radiographs are normal, but MRI shows bone oedema and stress fractures.

Diabetic foot ulcers are classified according to Wagner and Meggitt as follows:

Grade 0 – intact skin, but foot at risk
Grade 1 – localized superficial ulcer
Grade 2 – deep ulcer to tendon, bone or joint
Grade 3 – deep ulcer with abscess or osteomyelitis
Grade 4 – forefoot/toes gangrene
Grade 5 – whole foot gangrene

The Wagner and Meggitt classification has been superseded by Brodsky's alphanumeric classification of foot ulcers, which uses the numerals to describe the ulcer, and letters to describe the ischaemia.

9. 1. **h. Open repair**. 2. **g. Open reduction and internal fixation**. 3. **a. A non-weight-bearing, below knee cast**.

Traumatic dislocation of the peroneus brevis tendon is usually as a result of a dorsiflexion injury with reflex contraction of the peroneus brevis. Non-operative treatment of acute injuries in the young and active has a high recurrence rate (>50%), thus open repair, with or without deepening of the tendon groove, is advised. A lateral malleolar fracture with talar shift should be treated by open reduction and internal fixation. Subtalar dislocations are rare and may be associated with a tarsal fracture. Isolated dislocations, which are reducible, can be treated in a non-weight-bearing, below knee cast. On occasion, closed reduction is not possible as a result of soft tissue interposition. The structures blocking reduction are:

Medial dislocation – peroneal tendons, extensor digitorum brevis or talonavicular joint capsule

Lateral dislocation – tibialis posterior tendon, flexor hallucis longus or flexor digitorum longus

10. 1. **f. Flexor hallucis longus impingement**. 2. **j. Haglund's deformity**. 3. **e. Plantar fasciitis**.

Flexor hallucis longus impingement at the level of the posterior ankle joint causes posteromedial ankle pain. It is seen often in dancers. Non-operative treatment is often sufficient, although on occasions open or arthroscopic release at the ankle is required, with excision of an os trigonum or Stieda's process. A Haglund's deformity is a posterosuperior prominence of the calcaneal tuberosity, which can impinge on the Achilles tendon insertion and cause pain. Plantar fasciitis is a common cause of heel pain. The characteristic feature is medial heel pain, which is worse first thing in the morning, improves as the day goes on then worsens again in the evening. Treatment includes Achilles and local plantar fascial stretching, cushioning of the heel and night splints. Resistant cases may benefit from shockwave therapy or surgical release with plantar fasciotomy.

11. 1. **j. Fifth metatarsal**. 2. **i. First metatarsal**. 3. **i. First metatarsal**.

An accurate knowledge of muscle origins and attachments is important, not only to appreciate their function, but also to manage trauma and pathology. The peroneus brevis arises from the lower two-thirds of the lateral fibular shaft and inserts onto the tuberosity of the base of the fifth metatarsal. The peroneus longus arises from the upper third of the lateral fibular shaft, the fibular head and the proximal tibiofibular joint, and inserts onto the plantar aspect of the base of the first metatarsal and medial cuneiform. The tibialis anterior arises from the upper half of the lateral shaft of the tibia and interosseus membrane and inserts onto the inferomedial aspect of the medial cuneiform and base of the first metatarsal.

12. 1. **k. Lateral approach to the hindfoot (Ollier's)**. 2. **j. Posterior approach to the ankle**. 3. **h. Anterior approach to the ankle**.

Many approaches are available for the foot and ankle. Ollier's approach lies between peroneus tertius (deep peroneal nerve) and peroneus brevis (superficial peroneal nerve), and deeper involves detaching and reflecting extensor digitorum brevis. It exposes the subtalar, calcaneocuboid and talonavicular joints. It is largely historical as it risks dividing branches of the superficial peroneal nerve. The posterior approach to the ankle uses the interval between flexor hallucis longus (tibial nerve) and the peroneal muscles (superficial peroneal nerve). It is used to expose the posterior tibial margin, the fibula (in particular for an anti-glide plate), the ankle and subtalar joints. The anterior approach to the ankle is between the extensor hallucis longus and extensor digitorum longus, although this is not an internervous plane.

13. 1. **d. 11°**. 2. **e. 18°**. 3. **e. 18°**.
An appreciation of the grading of hallux valgus according to the hallux valgus angle (HVA) and intermetatarsal angle (IMA) is important, not only for orthopaedic examinations, but also in deciding treatment for the patient.

	HVA	IMA
Normal	<15°	<9°
Mild	15–19°	9–13°
Moderate	20–40°	14–20°
Severe	>40°	>20°

14. 1. **b. Anterior talofibular ligament**. 2. **b. Anterior talofibular ligament**.
  3. **a. Anterior-inferior tibiofibular ligament**.
The lateral ligament complex of the ankle comprises of the anterior talofibular ligament, calcaneo-fibular ligament and posterior talofibular ligament. The anterior talofibular ligament is the most commonly injured ligament and is the primary restraint to inversion in plantarflexion. The inferior tibiofibular joint (syndesmosis) is made up of the anterior-inferior tibiofibular ligament, posterior-inferior tibiofibular ligament, transverse tibiofibular ligament and interosseous ligament. Based on cadaveric studies, the percentage resistance to 2 mm of diastasis is 35% for the anterior-inferior tibiofibular ligament, 22% for the interosseous ligament, 9% for the posterior-inferior tibiofibular ligament and 33% for the transverse tibiofibular ligament.

15. 1. **d. Psoriatic arthropathy**. 2. **c. Ankylosing spondylitis**. 3. **g. Reiter's syndrome**.
A variety of systemic inflammatory conditions present with foot and ankle manifestations. Psoriatic arthropathy typically presents with dactylitis of a lesser toe. A 'sausage toe', with erythema and cylindrical enlargement is classical. Psoriatic arthropathy is an erosive arthritis and is associated with the 'pencil-in-cup' appearance of the distal interphalangeal joints of the hands and feet on radiographs. Ankylosing spondylitis, which is typically associated with back pain and stiffness, also causes enthesopathies such as plantar fasciitis and insertional Achilles tendinitis. Radiographs may show bony erosions at the origin of the plantar fascia. Reiter's syndrome classically presents with uveitis, arthritis and urethritis – hence the urological referral. Reiter's syndrome is a reactive arthritis to a preceding, or simultaneous, gastrointestinal or urological infection. It may present with insertional Achilles tendinitis; if ciprofloxacin has been used to treat the infection, this should be stopped as it may exacerbate the tendinitis and predispose to tendon rupture.

Selected references

Berndt AL, Harty M. Transchondral fractures (osteochondritis dissecans) of the talus. *J Bone Joint Surg Am* 1959; **41**: 988–1020.

Buck P, Morrey BF, Chao EY. The optimum position of arthrodesis of the ankle. A gait study of the knee and ankle. *J Bone Joint Surg Am* 1987; **69**(7): 1052–62.

Calder JD, Whitehouse SL, Saxby TS. Results of isolated Lisfranc injuries and the effect of compensation claims. *J Bone Joint Surg Br* 2004; **86**(4): 527–30.

Canale ST, Beaty JH. *Campbell's Operative Orthopaedics'* 11th edn. Philadelphia, Mosby, 2007.

Grayson ML, Gibbons GW, Balogh K, Levin E, Karchmer AW. Probing to bone in infected pedal ulcers: a clinical sign of underlying osteomyelitis in diabetic patients. *JAMA* 1995; **273**: 721–3.

Hoppenfeld S, deBoer P, Buckley R. *Surgical Exposures in Orthopaedics: The Anatomic Approach*, 3rd edn. Philadelphia, Lippincott Williams and Wilkins, 2009.

Khan RJ, Fick D, Keogh A *et al.* Treatment of acute Achilles tendon ruptures. A meta-analysis of randomized, controlled trials. *J Bone Joint Surg Am* 2005; **87**(10): 2202–10.

Miller MD. *Review of Orthopaedics*, 5th edn. Philadelphia, Elsevier, 2008.

Myerson MS, Fisher RT, Burgess AR, Kenzora JE. Fracture dislocations of the tarsometatarsal joints: end results correlated with pathology and treatment. *Foot Ankle* 1986; **6**: 225–42.

Ogilvie-Harris DJ, Reed SC, Hedman TP. Disruption of the ankle syndesmosis: biomechanical study of the ligamentous restraints. *Arthroscopy* 1994; **10**(5): 558–60.

Ramsey PL, Hamilton W. Changes in tibiotalar area of contact caused by lateral talar shift. *J Bone Joint Surg Am* 1976; **58**(3): 356–7.

Robinson AH, Limbers JP. Modern concepts in the treatment of hallux valgus. *J Bone Joint Surg Br* 2005; **87**(8): 1038–45.

Robinson AH, Pasapula C, Brodsky JW. Surgical aspects of the diabetic foot. *J Bone Joint Surg Br* 2009; **91**(1): 1–7.

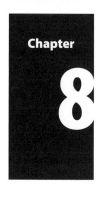

Pathology: Questions

Danyal H. Nawabi and Tim W.R. Briggs

MCQs

1. **A 12-year-old boy presents with a 2 month history of right knee pain after a fall. He has lost 3 kg in weight but is otherwise well. He is pale, apyrexial and his right knee is slightly swollen and warm on examination. Plain radiographs reveal areas of dense sclerosis admixed with areas of radiolucency in the distal femoral metaphysis. Aggressive periosteal new bone formation is also noted. Which of the following is the most likely diagnosis?**
   a. Parosteal osteosarcoma.
   b. Periosteal osteosarcoma.
   c. High-grade intramedullary osteosarcoma.
   d. Telangiectatic osteosarcoma.
   e. Osteomyelitis.

2. **Prognostic factors that adversely affect survival in osteosarcoma include expression of all of the following except?**
   a. Anti-shock protein 90 antibodies.
   b. Chemokine receptor type 4(CXCR-4).
   c. Alkaline phosphatase (ALP).
   d. Vascular endothelial growth factor (VEGF).
   e. P-glycoprotein.

3. **A 28-year-old female presents to your clinic with progressively increasing pain in her left wrist. She has also recently been having repeated episodes of abdominal discomfort, nausea and vomiting. A plain radiograph of the wrist reveals an eccentrically placed lytic lesion in the metaphysis and epiphysis with thinning of the cortex. You suspect a giant cell tumour of bone. What is the most appropriate next step in the management of this patient?**
   a. Perform a bone biopsy.
   b. Curettage alone.
   c. Curettage and phenolization.
   d. Curettage, high-speed burr, cement and bone graft.
   e. Check serum parathyroid hormone (PTH) and calcium.

Postgraduate Orthopaedics, ed. Kesavan Sri-Ram. Published by Cambridge University Press.
© Cambridge University Press 2012.

4. A 55-year-old male is diagnosed with a dedifferentiated chondrosarcoma of the femur which appears on MRI to have a significant extraosseous component. Distant staging has not revealed any metastases. What surgical stage would be assigned to this tumour according to the system of the Musculoskeletal Tumour Society (MSTS)?
   a. IA.
   b. IB.
   c. IIA.
   d. IIB.
   e. IIIB.

5. Which of the following describes the signal sequences on T1- and T2-weighted MRI imaging of a soft tissue sarcoma?
   a. High (T1)/Moderate (T2).
   b. Low (T1)/Moderate (T2).
   c. Low (T1)/Low (T2).
   d. Low (T1)/High (T2).
   e. High (T1)/Low (T2).

6. A 17-year-old boy presents with a haemarthrosis in the left knee. There is no history of trauma. His parents mention that they have recently noted their son having protracted bleeding from minor cuts. The patient also reports a long history of abdominal pain and diarrhoea. On examination, the patient is of short stature and appears emaciated. Abdominal examination is unremarkable but an anal fissure is noted. Blood tests show a microcytic anaemia with a prolonged prothrombin time (PT) and a prolonged activated partial thromboplastin time (APTT). Further evaluation of clotting factors is likely to show low levels of which of the following?
   a. Factors II, V, VII, IX and X.
   b. Factor VIII.
   c. Factor IX.
   d. von Willebrand factor.
   e. Factors II, VII, IX and X.

7. Which one of the following is not true of articular cartilage composition in severe osteoarthritis?
   a. Increased water content.
   b. Decreased chondroitin 4-sulphate concentration.
   c. Decreased collagen content.
   d. Decreased keratin sulphate:chondroitin sulphate ratio.
   e. Decreased modulus of elasticity.

8. A 10-year-old boy presents with difficulty rising from a crouching position. On examination he is noted to be obese, hypertensive and has multiple small bruises on his limbs. Which of the following investigations is most appropriate to yield the likely diagnosis?
   a. Thyroid function tests.
   b. Serum creatine phosphokinase and muscle biopsy.
   c. Urine cortisol.
   d. Serum glucose.
   e. MRI pituitary gland.

9. A 17-year-old boy sustains multiple fractures of his lower limbs during his first full season playing in the youth team for a premier league football club. On examination, he is noted to have hepatomegaly. Radiographs of his lower limbs show dense sclerosis of his femora and tibiae with enlarged flask-shaped metaphyses. Which one of the following statements is true with regard to the underlying diagnosis?
   a. The autosomal dominant form can lead to death in infancy.
   b. The number of osteoclasts are usually reduced.
   c. The disorder may result from a defect in the thyroid.
   d. The lacunae are characteristically empty.
   e. Albers-Schönberg disease is the autosomal recessive form.

10. All of the following are true of cat scratch disease except?
   a. The causative organism is *Pasteurella multocida*.
   b. The antibiotic of choice is azithromycin.
   c. Painful lymphadenitis is a feature.
   d. Aspiration of suppurative lymph nodes is acceptable treatment.
   e. Disease transmission is via a wound inflicted by a cat.

11. Vitamin D-resistant rickets is inherited as which of the following traits?
   a. Autosomal dominant.
   b. Autosomal recessive.
   c. X-linked dominant.
   d. X-linked recessive.
   e. Non-Mendelian.

12. A 27-year-old male presents with a 1 year history of progressive pain and swelling in the tibia. Examination reveals anterior bowing of the tibia. Radiographs show multiple well-circumscribed lucent lesions separated by sclerotic bone in the tibial diaphysis. Histology shows epithelial-like cells in a glandular pattern on a background of fibrous stroma. What is the recommended treatment for this condition?
   a. Close observation.
   b. Internal fixation and bone grafting.
   c. Chemotherapy, wide surgical resection and limb salvage.
   d. Wide surgical resection and limb salvage.
   e. Extracorporeal radiotherapy.

13. The diagnostic criteria for ankylosing spondylitis include all of the following except?
   a. HLA B27 positivity.
   b. Limitation of motion of the lumbar spine.
   c. History of pain in the lumbar spine.
   d. Limited chest expansion to 2.5 cm or less.
   e. Sacroiliac joint involvement.

14. Which of the following tumours is least likely to involve the posterior elements of the spine?
   a. Osteoid osteoma.
   b. Langerhans' cell histiocytosis.
   c. Aneurysmal bone cyst.

d. Osteoblastoma.

e. Osteochondroma.

15. **All of the following principles must be adhered to when performing a biopsy of a bone tumour except?**

a. The selection of the biopsy path should be made in consultation with the surgeon who will perform the definitive excision.

b. The biopsy tract should be marked to allow excision at the time of definitive surgery.

c. The biopsy should ideally be performed at the centre where the definitive excision is likely to be carried out.

d. The tumour should be approached through normal tissue before entering the reactive zone.

e. Use of frozen section to ensure that diagnostic tissue has been obtained.

16. **What is the World Health Organization (WHO) definition of osteoporosis?**

a. Bone mineral density less than 1 standard deviation below the mean of a young, healthy adult.

b. Bone mineral density at least 2.5 standard deviations below the mean of a young, healthy adult.

c. T score less than −2.5.

d. T score more than −2.5.

e. B and C.

17. **Curettage and grafting is acceptable treatment for all of the following lesions except?**

a. Osteoblastoma.

b. Aneurysmal bone cyst.

c. Osteofibrous dysplasia.

d. Chondromyxoid fibroma.

e. Fibrous dysplasia.

18. **A 30-year-old male presents with a bony growth arising from the proximal phalanx of his left middle finger which appeared 3 months ago and is steadily increasing in size, and now causing discomfort. He denies a history of trauma. Radiographs demonstrate an irregular bony mass arising from the dorsolateral surface of the proximal phalanx. The matrix of the lesion contains mature bone. What is the diagnosis?**

a. Osteochondroma.

b. Nora's disease.

c. Periosteal chondroma.

d. Parosteal osteosarcoma.

e. Myositis ossificans.

19. **Which one of the following benign tumours can metastasize to the lung?**

a. Osteoid osteoma.

b. Non-ossifying fibroma.

c. Haemangioma.

d. Eosinophilic granuloma.

e. Chondroblastoma.

20. **Which of the following lesions is least likely to affect the epiphysis?**
    a. Clear cell chondrosarcoma.
    b. Chondromyxoid fibroma.
    c. Giant cell tumour.
    d. Osteomyelitis.
    e. Chondroblastoma.

21. **Which of the following is not a feature of hypophosphatasia?**
    a. Decreased serum phosphate levels.
    b. Decreased alkaline phosphatase activity.
    c. Muscle hypotonia.
    d. Pathological fractures.
    e. Elevated urinary phosphoethanolamine.

22. **All of the following are features of giant cell tumour of bone except?**
    a. The most common site in the axial skeleton is the sacrum.
    b. Located in an eccentric position along the long axis of a bone.
    c. Cross the physis.
    d. Metastasize to lung.
    e. Metaphyseal–epiphyseal location.

23. **Which of the following conditions presents with brachydactyly?**
    a. Apert's syndrome.
    b. Poland's syndrome.
    c. Albright's hereditary osteodystrophy.
    d. Haemochromatosis.
    e. Hypoparathyroidism.

24. **A 70-year-old male presents with weight loss, fatigue and back pain. Examination reveals hepatomegaly and axillary lymphadenopathy. Blood tests show a raised calcium and erythrocyte sedimentation rate. Serum protein electrophoresis reveals an M-protein spike, with an elevated serum IgM level. Urinary Bence-Jones proteins are detected. Radiographs show lytic lesions in the T6, T8 and T9 vertebrae. These are cold on bone scan. Biopsy reveals intensely eosinophilic plasma cells. Which of the following is the most likely diagnosis?**
    a. Multiple myeloma.
    b. Plasmacytoma.
    c. POEMS (polyneuropathy, organomegaly, endocrinopathy, monoclonal gammopathy and skin changes) syndrome.
    d. Waldenström macroglobulinaemia.
    e. Monoclonal gammopathy of undetermined significance.

25. **Which of the following is true regarding Ollier's disease?**
    a. Autosomal dominant.
    b. Sarcomatous degeneration occurs in 30% of patients.
    c. Hand involvement is an uncommon feature.
    d. Incidence of conversion to chondrosarcoma is similar to Mafucci's syndrome.
    e. Onset is usually in adulthood.

26. All of the following are features of McCune–Albright syndrome except?
    a. 'Coast of Maine' café-au-lait patches.
    b. Precocious puberty.
    c. Ground glass appearance.
    d. Woven bone without osteoblastic rimming.
    e. Mutation of the Gi alpha subunit of a membrane G protein.

27. The commonest cause for a Charcot's arthropathy in the upper limb is?
    a. Hansen's disease.
    b. Myelomeningocele.
    c. Diabetes.
    d. Tabes dorsalis.
    e. Syringomyelia.

28. A 31-year-old male presents with stiffness and pain in his back and hips.
    Examination reveals a bluish-grey discolouration of his ear cartilage and sclera
    and decreased range of movement in his hips. His urine is noted to be black.
    Radiographs of his lumbar spine show multilevel disc degeneration. This patient
    most likely has a deficiency of which of the following enzymes?
    a. Muscle phosphorylase.
    b. Hexosaminidase A.
    c. Cystathione β-synthase.
    d. Homogentisic acid oxidase.
    e. β-galactosidase.

29. A 2-year-old infant presents with seizures and hair loss. He is noted to have a positive
    Chvostek's sign and an electrocardiogram shows a prolonged QT interval. His
    parents say that he has also suffered from multiple infections since birth due to a
    T-cell deficiency. This child's syndrome is associated with failure of the
    development of which of the following embryonic structures?
    a. Neural crest.
    b. Third and fourth pharyngeal pouches.
    c. Rathke's pouch.
    d. Foramen caecum.
    e. Urogenital ridge.

30. Which one of the following is not a diagnostic criterion for rheumatoid arthritis
    according to the American Rheumatism Association?
    a. Raised rheumatoid factor.
    b. Symmetric swelling (arthritis) for at least 6 weeks.
    c. Symmetrical muscle weakness.
    d. Rheumatoid nodules.
    e. Positive radiographic changes.

EMQs

1. Laboratory findings in metabolic bone disease

	Ca	Phos	ALP	PTH	25-hydroxy vitamin D	1,25 dihydroxy vitamin D	Urinary Ca
a.	L	H	H	H	N	L	L
b.	H	L	H	H	N	N	H
c.	L	H	N	H	N	L	L
d.	L	L	H	H	H	H	L
e.	H	H	L	N	N	N	H
f.	N	L	H	N	N	N	H
g.	L	L	H	H	H	L	L

Which one of the options above is best described in each of the following statements? Each option may be used once, more than once or not at all.
1. This is the most commonly encountered form of rickets.
2. A 67-year-old patient on haemodialysis who is also noted to have 'brown tumours' in his skeleton.
3. A young patient who has total baldness with an autosomal recessive form of rickets. The defective enzyme produces the active form of vitamin D.

2. Haematological disorders encountered in orthopaedics
a. Bernard–Soulier syndrome
b. Von Willebrand disease
c. Thrombotic thrombocytopaenic purpura
d. Idiopathic thrombocytopaenic purpura
e. Factor V Leiden deficiency
f. Haemophilia A
g. Christmas disease
h. Henoch–Schonlein purpura
i. Heparin-induced thrombocytopaenia
j. Paroxysmal nocturnal haemoglobinuria

Which one of the options above is best described in each of the following statements? Each option may be used once, more than once or not at all.
1. A 15-year-old boy presents with a 45 minute history of persistent bleeding after sustaining an abrasion around his knee while playing football. He is noted to have scattered petechiae across his body. His clotting profile reveals a normal platelet count with no elevation in prothrombin time (PT) or activated partial thromboplastin time (APTT), but a prolonged bleeding time.
2. This bleeding disorder is also characterized by a raised bleeding time and a normal platelet count, but does not respond to a platelet transfusion.
3. A 33-year-old male suffers from repeated haemarthroses of his knees and ankles and is currently awaiting a right ankle arthrodesis for severe degenerative change and deformity. He has a deficiency of factor IX.

3. **Genetic diseases linked to enzyme deficiencies presenting with orthopaedic problems**
   a. Niemann–Pick disease
   b. von Gierke disease
   c. Tay–Sachs disease
   d. Gaucher's disease
   e. McArdle syndrome
   f. Hunter's syndrome
   g. Hurler's syndrome
   h. Fabry disease
   i. Krabbe disease
   j. Lesch–Nyhan syndrome
   k. Morquio's syndrome

Which one of the options above is best described in each of the following statements? Each option may be used once, more than once or not at all.
   1. A 28-year-old male decides to start training for the London Marathon. He is otherwise fit and well but has not exercised much in the past. After his first training session he develops extremely painful muscle cramps in his quadriceps which he has not experienced before. He ensures that he hydrates himself adequately, but the cramps continue to trouble him in subsequent training sessions. He also notices that his urine has turned red.
   2. A 9-year-old boy of Jewish descent presents with a progressive limp. On examination he is noted to be extremely lethargic, has multiple bruises and has massive hepatosplenomegaly. His right hip joint is irritable and movements are limited because of pain.
   3. A 10-month-old male infant is brought to hospital by his parents as they are concerned about their son having weak limbs, being in pain and repeatedly biting his hands and lips. The mother mentions that she has noticed tiny, orange-coloured particles when she changes her son's diapers.

4. **Radiology of benign bone tumours**
   a. Osteoblastoma
   b. Osteoid osteoma
   c. Giant cell tumour
   d. Osteochondroma
   e. Chondromyxoid fibroma
   f. Chondroblastoma
   g. Non-ossifying fibroma
   h. Haemangioma
   i. Desmoplastic fibroma
   j. Enchondroma

Which one of the options above is most applicable to each of the following statements? Each option may be used once, more than once or not at all.
   1. A plain radiograph of the lumbar spine shows thickened vertical trabeculae of the L2 vertebra.
   2. A plain radiograph shows a sessile lesion arising from the distal clavicle. The cavity of the lesion is continuous with the medullary cavity of the clavicle.

151

3. A plain radiograph shows a lytic, destructive lesion in the metaphysis of the distal tibia. The lesion extends into the epiphysis but does not extend beyond the subchondral bone. Cortical thinning and breakthrough is noted.

5. **Immunology**
   a. DiGeorge syndrome
   b. Wiskott–Aldrich syndrome
   c. Complement factors
   d. IgA
   e. IgE
   f. IgG
   g. IgM
   h. Chronic granulomatous disease
   i. Type I hypersensitivity
   j. Type III hypersensitivity
   k. Type IV hypersensitivity

Which one of the options above is most applicable to each of the following statements? Each option may be used once, more than once or not at all.
1. A 24-year-old female is involved in a road traffic accident and sustains an open, comminuted femoral shaft fracture. She undergoes debridement and femoral nailing and requires four units of blood transfusion of the appropriate ABO and Rh type. As the transfusion progresses, she becomes hypotensive and goes into anaphylactic shock.
2. A 45-year-old female presents 1 year after having a right hip resurfacing with a painful right hip. After thorough investigation, metal allergy is considered as a possible diagnosis. She undergoes skin patch testing and is found to be allergic to nickel, amongst other metals.
3. A 20-year-old female presents with pain and tenosynovitis of her wrists and a very painful right knee and ankle. She has had one previous episode. She is otherwise well and completed her last menstrual period 3 days ago. Examination reveals ulcerated lesions over her wrists and ankles.

6. **Conditions mimicking bone tumours**
   a. Myositis ossificans
   b. Melorheostosis
   c. Pigmented villonodular synovitis (PVNS)
   d. Synovial chondromatosis
   e. Fibrous dysplasia
   f. Paget's disease
   g. Nora's disease
   h. Bone island
   i. Tumoral calcinosis
   j. Aneurysmal bone cyst
   k. Unicameral bone cyst

Which one of the options above is most applicable to each of the following statements? Each option may be used once, more than once or not at all.
1. A 13-year-old boy presents with knee pain after an injury sustained while playing football. Examination does not reveal any evidence of ligamentous incompetence.

A plain radiograph shows a cystic lesion in the proximal tibial metaphysis with no fracture. An MRI scan shows multiple fluid lines within the lesion.

2. A 35-year-old Afro-Caribbean male presents with a 2 year history of right hip pain. Movements of the right hip are minimally restricted and there is a non-tender fullness palpable in the right buttock. Radiographs show multiple, well-demarcated, calcified deposits around the right hip joint.

3. A 55-year-old male presents to the clinic with an arthritic hip. His radiographs confirm osteoarthritis of his hip and also show very thickened femoral cortices which in some parts of the femur almost completely obliterate the medullary cavity. When performing his hip replacement, the surgeon encounters extreme difficulty when trying to prepare the femoral canal.

7. **Histological features of bone tumours**
   a. 'Birbeck' granules
   b. 'Storiform' pattern
   c. 'Foamy' physaliferous cells
   d. 'Alphabet soup' pattern
   e. 'Herringbone' pattern
   f. 'Lacey' osteoid
   g. 'Clock face' pattern
   h. 'Chicken wire' calcification
   i. 'Biphasic' pattern

Which one of the options above is most applicable to each of the following statements? Each option may be used once, more than once or not at all.

1. A 9-year-old boy presents with painless bowing of the tibia. On examination he has mild tenderness over the most prominent aspect of the anterior surface of the tibia. His radiographs show an anterior eccentric lesion confined to the anterior cortex of the tibia. A procurvatum deformity of the tibia is noted.

2. A 62-year-old female presents with pain and swelling in her left arm. The patient is noted to have exophthalmus. Radiographs show a lytic lesion in the humeral diaphysis with well-defined margins.

3. A 12-year-old boy presents with 2 months of increasing pain in his right shoulder. It is particularly bad at night. He lacks full abduction and external rotation because of pain. Radiographs reveal a well-circumscribed epiphyseal lytic lesion with a thin rim of sclerotic bone.

8. **Mechanism of action of antibiotics used in orthopaedics**
   a. Aminoglycosides
   b. Penicillins
   c. Cephalosporins
   d. Clindamycin
   e. Imipenem/Meropenem
   f. Vancomycin
   g. Tetracyclines
   h. Macrolides
   i. Fluoroquinolones

    j. Rifampicin
    k. Trimethoprim
    l. Linezolid

Which one of the options above is best described in each of the following statements? Each option may be used once, more than once or not at all.

1. Inhibits DNA-dependent RNA polymerase and can give red-orange urine.
2. Blocks the attachment of aminoacyl-tRNA to the acceptor site on the 30S ribosomal subunit, thus preventing prokaryotic protein synthesis.
3. Works as an antimetabolite by inhibiting dihydrofolate reductase.

9. **Organisms in orthopaedics**
    a. Methicillin-resistant *Staphylococcus aureus*
    b. *Pseudomonas aeruginosa*
    c. *Brucella*
    d. *Bartonella henselae*
    e. *Staphylococcus epidermidis*
    f. *Peptostreptococcus*
    g. *Borrelia burgdorferi*
    h. *Candida albicans*
    i. *Treponema pallidum*
    j. *Nocardia*
    k. *Vibrio vulnificus*
    l. *Streptococcus viridans*
    m. *Pasteurella multocida*
    n. *Eikenella corrodens*

Which one of the options above is best described in each of the following statements? Each option may be used once, more than once or not at all.

1. A 56-year-old female has recently had a dental procedure. She presents with an infected total hip replacement which was performed 11 years ago.
2. A 24-year-old male presents to the emergency department with a 'fight bite' wound over the middle finger metacarpal.
3. A 45-year-old male presents a red rash on his back and an effusion in his shoulder. The causative organism is transmitted by the Ixodes tick.

10. **Osteomyelitis**
    a. Acute haematogenous osteomyelitis
    b. Subacute osteomyelitis
    c. Brodie's abscess
    d. Garre's sclerosing osteomyelitis
    e. Multifocal osteomyelitis
    f. Tuberculous osteomyelitis
    g. Epiphyseal osteomyelitis
    h. Contiguous-focus osteomyelitis
    i. Chronic osteomyelitis
    j. B, C

Which one of the options above is best described in each of the following statements? Each option may be used once, more than once or not at all.

1. An otherwise fit and well 11-year-old boy presents with a 3 month history of pain in his left tibia and right clavicle. There is no history of trauma. The affected bones are tender and warm to touch. Blood tests are normal apart from an elevated erythrocyte sedimentation rate (ESR). Radiographs show radiolucent lesions in the tibia and clavicle with radiodense borders and minimal periosteal reaction.

2. A 7-year-old girl presents with a 6 month history of a progressively painful limp. There is no history of trauma. She is systemically well and has mild tenderness over the lateral aspect of the right femur. White blood cell count, ESR and C-reactive protein (CRP) are normal. Radiographs reveal a localized radiolucency in the right distal femoral metaphysis with surrounding sclerosis.

3. A 17-year-old male presents with intense pain in his right lower leg, after recovering from a recent infection of his right first molar. Localized tenderness is noted over the midshaft of the right tibia. Radiographs show an 'onion-skin' appearance of the tibial diaphysis. A biopsy rules out malignancy, but shows the presence of anaerobes.

11. **Management of bone tumours**
    a. Observe
    b. Prophylactic stabilization
    c. Curettage and grafting
    d. Radiotherapy
    e. Chemotherapy
    f. Hormonal therapy
    g. Angiographic embolization
    h. Radiotherapy and wide excision
    i. Neoadjuvant chemotherapy and wide excision
    j. Massive endoprosthetic replacement
    k. Non-invasive grower
    l. Extracorporeal radiotherapy
    m. Amputation
    n. I and J
    o. I and K

Which one of the options above is best described in each of the following statements? Each option may be used once, more than once or not at all.

1. A 28-year-old female presents with a recurrent giant cell tumour of bone in her right index finger metacarpal. She has had two previous attempts at aggressive intralesional curettage. MRI confirms recurrent disease with a very large soft tissue component. A CT scan of her chest does not show any evidence of lung metastasis.

2. A 55-year-old male presents with a 4 month history of pain in his right lower leg. He has a previous history of a nephrectomy for renal cell carcinoma. After routine investigation, he is diagnosed with a solitary renal metastasis in the diaphysis of his right fibula.

3. A 10-year-old boy presents with knee pain, fever and swelling around the knee. He is diagnosed with a Ewing's sarcoma of the distal femur with no evidence of metastases.

12. **Genetics in orthopaedic oncology**
    a. pRB-1
    b. p53
    c. erb-B2
    d. N-myc
    e. t (11:22)
    f. t (2:13)
    g. t (12:16)
    h. t (X:18)
    i. t (12:22)
    j. t (9:22)
    k. EXT1 and EXT2

Which one of the options above is best described in each of the following statements? Each option may be used once, more than once or not at all.
1. A 19-year-old female presents with a mass in the foot. She is diagnosed with the most common sarcoma found in the foot.
2. An 8-year-old girl has an autosomal recessive condition which has caused blindness in one eye. She presents with pain and swelling in her left knee.
3. An 18-year-old boy presents with a painful lump on his right thigh. He is diagnosed with a sarcoma. The histology shows 'racquet-shaped' cells and immunostaining is vimentin positive.

13. **Inflammatory arthritides and connective tissue disorders**
    a. Rheumatoid arthritis
    b. Systemic lupus erythematosus (SLE)
    c. Ankylosing spondylitis
    d. Disseminated idiopathic skeletal hyperostosis (DISH)
    e. Psoriatic arthritis
    f. Reiter's syndrome
    g. Gout
    h. Pseudogout
    i. Sjögren's syndrome
    j. CREST syndrome
    k. Systemic sclerosis

Which one of the options above is best described in each of the following statements? Each option may be used once, more than once or not at all.
1. A 37-year-old female presents with fatigue and tender, swollen joints. Examination reveals a significant maculopapular eruption over the sun-exposed areas on her face. Blood tests show that she is positive for anti-Sm antibody.
2. A 50-year-old obese male presents with an acutely painful knee. Examination reveals an effusion. Radiographs show punched-out periarticular erosions.
3. A 60-year-old female presents with taut facial skin and peripheral cyanosis. She has long spindle-shaped fingers. Blood tests show that she is positive for anti-centromere antibody.

14. **Osteochondroses**
    a. Freiberg's disease
    b. Kienbock's disease
    c. Kohler's disease
    d. Sinding-Larsen–Johansson syndrome
    e. Van Neck's disease
    f. Sever's disease
    g. Thiemann's disease
    h. Panner's disease

Which one of the options above is best described in each of the following statements? Each option may be used once, more than once or not at all.
    1. A 9-year-old girl presents with posterolateral elbow pain and clicking.
    2. A 12-year-old boy presents with a limp after a fall from height. Examination reveals tenderness on the plantar aspect of the calcaneum.
    3. A 5-year-old boy presents with pain on walking. Examination reveals tenderness on the medial aspect of his foot.

15. **Anticoagulants**
    a. Unfractionated heparin
    b. Aspirin
    c. Warfarin
    d. Low-molecular-weight heparin
    e. Rivaroxaban
    f. Dabigatran
    g. Dextran

Which one of the options above is best described in each of the following statements? Each option may be used once, more than once or not at all.
    1. The dose of this drug may need to be increased when administered concomitantly with rifampicin.
    2. Orally active, direct factor Xa inhibitor.
    3. Thrombin inhibitor.

Pathology: Answers

Danyal H. Nawabi and Tim W.R. Briggs

MCQs

1. c. High-grade intramedullary osteosarcoma.

This vignette gives the classical presentation of osteosarcoma. The most common type of osteosarcoma is high-grade intramedullary osteosarcoma and usually occurs about the knee in adolescents and young adults. The primary presenting complaint is pain. Osteosarcomas are spindle cell neoplasms that produce osteoid. There are many types of osteosarcoma. Parosteal osteosarcoma often presents as a painless mass. It is low grade, tends to occur on the posterior surface of the distal femur and is more common in females. Periosteal osteosarcoma is a rare surface form of osteosarcoma which most often occurs in the diaphysis of long bones. Telangiectatic osteosarcoma is highly malignant and radiographically mimics aneurysmal bone cysts.

2. a. Anti-shock protein 90 antibodies.

The absence, not the expression, of anti-shock protein 90 antibodies after chemotherapy for osteosarcoma, is an adverse prognostic factor. The expression of CXCR-4 (chemotaxis marker), ALP, VEGF (vascular invasion marker) and P-glycoprotein (confers drug resistance to doxorubicin) adversely affect survival in osteosarcoma.

3. e. Check serum parathyroid hormone (PTH) and calcium.

This vignette highlights the issue of undiagnosed hyperparathyroidism presenting with a lytic lesion that can be mistaken for a giant cell tumour. The skeletal effects of hyperparathyroidism include massive bone resorption, bone fractures, bone pain, diffuse osteopaenia, or circumscribed lytic lesions. These lesions are referred to as 'brown tumours' and are radiologically and histologically similar to giant cell tumours. Clinically, hyperparathyroidism presents as 'bones, stones, groans and moans'. The patient in this case has bone pain 'bones' and gastrointestinal symptoms 'groans'. This should prompt the consideration of hyperparathyroidism as a diagnosis. A simple blood test looking for a raised serum calcium and PTH will confirm the diagnosis and avoid the need for a potentially unnecessary biopsy. Choices B, C and D should not be considered until a diagnosis is established. The treatment of 'brown tumours' is dependent upon the underlying aetiology of the hyperparathyroidism.

Postgraduate Orthopaedics, ed. Kesavan Sri-Ram. Published by Cambridge University Press.
© Cambridge University Press 2012.

4. **d. IIB.**

The case in this question is of a high-grade tumour (dedifferentiated chondrosarcoma), which has invaded its natural anatomical barrier (periosteum) to become extraosseous and hence extracompartmental, in the absence of metastases, i.e. stage IIB.

Stage is determined by three different subcategories:

1. Grade (histology with aid of radiographic findings and clinical correlation)

   G1: Low grade
   G2: High grade

2. Site

   T1: Intracompartmental
   T2: Extracompartmental

3. Metastasis

   M0: No identifiable skip lesions or distant metastases
   M1: Any skip lesions, regional lymph nodes or distant metastases

Enneking's and MSTS Staging System of Malignant Bone Tumours:

IA	Low grade, intracompartmental	G1	T1	M0
IB	Low grade, extracompartmental	G1	T2	M0
IIA	High grade, intracompartmental	G2	T1	M0
IIB	High grade, extracompartmental	G2	T2	M0
IIIA	Any grade, intracompartmental, with metastases	G1/2	T1	M1
IIIB	Any grade, extracompartmental, with metastases	G1/2	T2	M1

5. **d. Low (T1)/High (T2).**

MRI uses radiofrequency pulses on tissues in a magnetic field to generate images in different planes. Protons in compounds of hydrogen (e.g. water, fat, marrow, etc) are aligned in a magnetic field. The strength of this imaging modality is its sensitivity to changes in water distribution. T1 images are weighted towards fat and T2 images are weighted towards water. Water, cerebrospinal fluid and soft tissue tumours appear dark on T1 sequences and bright on T2 sequences. Fat, nerves and bone marrow appear bright on T1 sequences and grey (moderate) on T2 sequences.

6. **e. Factors II, VII, IX and X.**

This case requires an understanding of the clotting cascade and knowledge of which factors would cause an elevation of both the PT and APTT. For both of these times to be elevated, a deficiency of clotting factors involved in both the extrinsic and intrinsic pathways is required. This narrows down the choices to either A or E. The patient in this case has Crohn's disease. This can affect the terminal ileum resulting in malabsorption of the fat-soluble vitamins A, D, E and K. Factors II, VII, IX and X are the vitamin K-dependent clotting factors, which would be expected to be low in Crohn's disease. Factor V would also be low if the patient had liver disease but this is not stated in the vignette.

Factor VIII deficiency is the cause of haemophilia A. This would give an elevated APTT but a normal PT. Factor IX deficiency is the cause of Christmas disease, which is again characterized by an elevated APTT but a normal PT. Low levels of von Willebrand factor are seen in von Willebrand disease. This causes a prolonged or normal APTT, a normal PT and a prolonged bleeding time.

7. b.   Decreased chondroitin 4-sulphate concentration.
Chondroitin sulphate concentration increases in osteoarthritis and this includes both chondroitin 4- and 6-sulphate. Keratin sulphate concentration decreases and hence the ratio of keratin to chondroitin sulphate decreases as well.

8. c.   Urine cortisol.
The opening line of this case may tempt one to consider the diagnosis of Duchenne's muscular dystrophy for which choice B would be the correct answer. This child has features of Cushing's syndrome, which can be caused by excess adrenocorticotrophic hormone (ACTH) production or occur independent of ACTH, due to an adrenal adenoma. Obesity, hypertension, bruising and proximal myopathy are all features of Cushing's syndrome. The first step in establishing this diagnosis is to measure the urinary free cortisol. The cause of the Cushing's syndrome can then be determined by performing the dexamethasone suppression test, measuring plasma ACTH and obtaining an MRI of the pituitary if appropriate.

9. d.   The lacunae are characteristically empty.
This patient has osteopetrosis. This bone disorder is characterized by increased sclerosis and obliteration of the medullary canals secondary to decreased osteoclast function and not number. Pathological fractures are common. It may result from a thymic defect. Histologically, osteoclasts lack their normal brush border and empty lacunae with plugged Haversian canals are seen. The autosomal recessive form can lead to death during infancy and the autosomal dominant form (Albers-Schönberg disease) tends to have a more benign course.

10. a.   The causative organism is *Pasteurella multocida*.
Cat scratch disease is caused by a wound inflicted by a cat. It causes infection of the lymphatic system by *Bartonella henselae*. Treatment can be supportive as the disease resolves in 2–6 months. Symptomatic treatment in the form of aspiration of painful lymph nodes is acceptable. Incision and drainage of these nodes is contraindicated. The antibiotic of choice is azithromycin. *Pasteurella multocida* is the causative organism in cat bite injuries.

11. c.   X-linked dominant.
Vitamin D-resistant rickets is also known as familial hypophosphataemic rickets. It is an X-linked dominant disorder that occurs as a result of renal phosphate wasting. It is the most common form of rickets and is treated with phosphate replacement.

12. d.   Wide surgical resection and limb salvage.
This patient has an adamantinoma. This is an extremely rare, low-grade, malignant tumour of long bones. It is almost always found on the anterior cortex of the tibia. It must be differentiated from osteofibrous dysplasia which also occurs on the anterior cortex of the

tibia, but tends to occur in children and is a benign condition. Adamantinoma is treated with wide surgical excision. It is not sensitive to radiotherapy, and chemotherapy is not used.

13. a. HLA B27 positivity.

Modified New York Criteria for diagnosing ankylosing spondylitis:

- Clinical criteria:

  Low back pain; present for more than 3 months; improved by exercise but not relieved by rest.
  Limitation of lumbar spine motion in both the sagittal and frontal planes.
  Limitation of chest expansion relative to normal values for age and sex.

- Radiological criterion:

  Sacroiliitis on X-ray.

- Diagnose:

  Definite ankylosing spondylitis if the radiological criterion is present plus at least one clinical criterion.
  Probable ankylosing spondylitis if three clinical criteria are present alone, or if the radiological criterion is present but no clinical criteria are present.

14. b. Langerhans' cell histiocytosis.

Langerhans' cell histiocytosis or eosinophilic granuloma is usually seen in the vertebral bodies of children and adolescents. The vertebral body tends to collapse producing the classical radiographic appearance of 'vertebra plana'. Rarely do these tumours lead to paraparesis and typically heal spontaneously.

15. d. The tumour should be approached through normal tissue before entering the reactive zone.

When performing a biopsy of a suspected bone tumour the following principles must be followed (in addition to A, B, C, E):

- avoid contamination of normal compartments
- enter the tumour through the reactive zone
- place the biopsy tract in line with incision to allow excision when performing a longitudinal extensile incision
- avoid contamination of intermuscular planes
- avoid contamination of neurovascular bundles

16. e. B and C.

In 1994, the WHO introduced definitions for osteoporosis and osteopaenia in terms of T score thresholds of –2.5 and –1 respectively. A T score of –2.5 means that the bone mineral density in the lumbar spine (L2–L4) is at least 2.5 standard deviations below the mean of a young (age 25–35), healthy female. A T score of more than –2.5 implies it is more positive and hence could represent either osteopaenia or normal bone density.

17. c. Osteofibrous dysplasia.

Most orthopaedic oncology centres would agree that there is no role for curettage and grafting in osteofibrous dysplasia. This condition often regresses by the time a child reaches skeletal maturity and therefore observation is all that is required. This line of management is controversial. Osteofibrous dysplasia has been linked to progression to adamantinoma, in which case wide surgical excision is recommended.

18. b. Nora's disease.
This patient has a bizarre parosteal osteochondromatous proliferation (BPOP). This is a rare lesion that tends to occur in the hands and feet and is thought to be related to myositis ossificans. It was first described in 1983 by Dr Nora; hence the name Nora's disease. The lesion is benign but may recur locally in up to 50% of cases. Recommended treatment is complete excision with the widest possible margin without damage to adjacent structures.

19. e. Chondroblastoma.
Benign skeletal tumours rarely if ever metastasize to lung. The two exceptions to this rule are giant cell tumour (up to 10% metastasize to lung) and chondroblastoma.

20. b. Chondromyxoid fibroma.
Helms has stated that 99% of epiphyseal lesions in young patients are one of the following: chondroblastoma, giant cell tumour, osteomyelitis, aneurysmal bone cyst and eosinophilic granuloma. Clear cell chondrosarcoma can also affect the epiphysis, but in an older age group. Chondromyxoid fibroma typically produces a lytic lesion in the metaphysis.

21. a. Decreased serum phosphate levels.
Hypophosphatasia is an autosomal recessive disorder caused by an inborn error of the isoenzyme of alkaline phosphatase (ALP). Its features are similar to those of rickets. It is not associated with decreased serum levels of phosphate or calcium. Vitamin D and parathyroid hormone (PTH) levels are usually normal.

22. c. Cross the physis.
Giant cell tumour of bone occurs in young adults aged 25–40. The physis must be closed for the radiological criteria to be met which are: 1. Epiphyseal location, 2. Abut the articular surface, 3. Eccentric, 4. Non-sclerotic margin. The most common sites in the appendicular skeleton are the distal femur and distal radius. The sacrum is the commonest site in the axial skeleton.

23. c. Albright's hereditary osteodystrophy.
Brachydactyly refers to short first, fourth and fifth metacarpals and metatarsals. This is seen in pseudohypoparathyroidism, otherwise known as Albright's hereditary osteodystrophy. This disorder occurs due to a parathyroid hormone (PTH) receptor abnormality. In addition to the brachydactyly, patients are obese, have reduced intelligence and can present with exostoses.

24. d. Waldenström macroglobulinaemia.
This question really requires you to read the vignette carefully. There are a number of clues that should prevent you from going straight for multiple myeloma (MM) as the answer. Firstly, the age of the patient. Peak incidence for Waldenström macroglobulinaemia (WM)

is 60–70 whereas for MM it is 50–60. The M spike in WM is IgM whereas in MM it is usually IgG. The intensely eosinophilic plasma cells are classic for WM. The multiple lesions rule out a solitary plasmacytoma. Patients with a monoclonal gammopathy of undetermined significance are asymptomatic. Patients with POEMS have symmetrical neurology and skin lesions.

25. b. Sarcomatous degeneration occurs in 30% of patients.
Ollier's disease is a non-inherited disease characterized by multiple enchondromas. Onset is usually in childhood and results in bony deformity and shortening. The lesions continue to progress until skeletal maturity. The risk of conversion to chondrosarcoma is 25–30% in Ollier's disease and up to 100% in Mafucci's syndrome.

26. e. Mutation of the Gi alpha subunit of a membrane G protein.
McCune–Albright syndrome is a condition defined by the presence of café-au-lait patches, precocious puberty and polyostotic fibrous dysplasia. Fibrous dysplasia has a ground glass appearance on plain radiographs and histologically features woven bone which lacks osteoblastic rimming. It arises due to a genetic mutation in the Gs alpha subunit (not the Gi subunit, which may have the opposite effect!) of a membrane G protein involved in cell signalling via the cAMP second messenger pathway.

27. e. Syringomyelia.
A Charcot's arthropathy is an extreme form of osteoarthritis caused by disturbed sensory innervation. Syringomyelia is the most common cause for an upper limb Charcot joint. Tabes dorsalis used to be the most common cause for a lower limb Charcot joint, but now diabetes is the most common cause.

28. d. Homogentisic acid oxidase.
This patient has degenerative arthritis resulting from alkaptonuria. This condition is also known as ochronosis. The deficient enzyme is homogentisic acid oxidase. Homogentisic acid is deposited in joints and turns black. It is also responsible for the black urine.

29. b. Third and fourth pharyngeal pouches.
This child has DiGeorge syndrome. The third pharyngeal pouch gives rise to the thymus and inferior parathyroid glands. The fourth pharyngeal pouch gives rise to the superior parathyroid glands. These patients therefore develop symptoms and signs of hypocalcaemia due to hypoparathyroidism and recurrent infections due to a T-cell deficiency which arises from inadequate development of the thymus. Other associations include tetralogy of Fallot, abnormal facies and cleft palate.

30. c. Symmetrical muscle weakness.
Rheumatoid arthritis is defined by the presence of four or more of the following criteria according to the American Rheumatism Association:
1. Morning stiffness in and around joints lasting at least 1 hour before maximal improvement, present for at least 6 weeks
2. Soft tissue swelling (arthritis) of three or more joint areas observed by a physician, present for at least 6 weeks

3. Swelling (arthritis) of the proximal interphalangeal, metacarpophalangeal or wrist joints for at least 6 weeks
4. Symmetric swelling (arthritis) for at least 6 weeks
5. Rheumatoid nodules
6. The presence of rheumatoid factor
7. Radiographic erosions and/or periarticular osteopaenia in hand and/or wrist joints

EMQs

1. 1. | f. | N | L | H | N | N | N | H |
   2. | a. | L | H | H | H | N | L | L |
   3. | g. | L | L | H | H | H | L | L |

The most commonly encountered form of rickets is familial hypophosphataemic rickets or vitamin D-resistant rickets. The kidney is unable to reabsorb phosphate resulting in phosphaturia and a low serum phosphate.

The 67-year-old patient has renal osteodystrophy. Renal disease impairs excretion of phosphate which lowers serum calcium and causes secondary hyperparathyroidism. Phosphorus also impairs renal 1α hydroxylase activity, thereby reducing production of 1,25 dihydroxy vitamin D.

The young patient has type I vitamin D-dependent rickets. This is due to a defect in renal 1α hydroxylase activity. It results in lowered levels of 1,25 dihydroxy vitamin D which in turn results in low calcium and high PTH levels.

The remainder of the profiles are of the following conditions:

B = Primary hyperparathyroidism, C = Pseudohyperparathyroidism, D = type II vitamin D-dependent rickets, E = Hypophosphatasia.

2. 1. **a. Bernard–Soulier syndrome.** 2. **b. Von Willebrand disease.** 3. **g. Christmas disease.** Bernard–Soulier syndrome is an autosomal recessive disease of platelet adhesion. The platelets cannot bind to subendothelial collagen due to dysfunction of the glycoprotein Ib–IX complex. A transfusion of normal platelets during an acute episode resolves the dysfunction in haemostasis.

Von Willebrand disease is caused by a defect in von Willebrand factor which aids the binding of platelets to collagen. The patients' platelets are inherently normal as opposed to Bernard–Soulier syndrome, but binding is impaired. Platelet transfusion does not therefore correct the problem. Cryoprecipitate, a plasma fraction rich in von Willebrand factor, resolves the acute bleeding episode.

Haemophilia B or Christmas disease is an X-linked recessive disorder characterized by repeated haemarthroses, particularly of the knee joint. Treatment of the underlying cause is addressed by factor replacement. For haemophiliacs requiring surgery, factor levels should be maintained near 100% during the first post-operative week and at 75% during the second week.

3. 1. **e. McArdle syndrome.** 2. **d. Gaucher's disease.** 3. **j. Lesch–Nyhan syndrome.** The first history is typical for the glycogen storage disease known as McArdle syndrome. Patients with this condition are deficient in muscle phosphorylase and accumulate glycogen in skeletal muscle. Glucose production and therefore energy supply in their muscles is impaired and they present with muscle weakness. Clinical onset is usually in the third decade and myoglobinuria may occur. The situation can be improved by drinking a sucrose-rich drink, which provides dietary glucose for the muscles to generate energy.

The second patient has Gaucher's disease. It is a lysosomal storage disease caused by a deficiency in the enzyme β-glucocerebrosidase. Glucocerebroside is a sphingolipid which is released when membrane is degraded and digested in endosomes after fusion with lysosomes. It arises mainly from the breakdown of old red and white blood cells. In the absence of β-glucocerebrosidase, glucocerebroside accumulates in cells and tissues responsible for its turnover. Histologically, this results in lipid-laden histiocytes, known as 'Gaucher' cells, which have a 'wrinkled-paper' cytoplasm. There are three clinical types of the disease. Type I is the most common, type II is infantile and type III is chronic neuropathic. Type I is most commonly seen in children of Ashkenazi Jewish descent. Its orthopaedic manifestations include osteopaenia, avascular necrosis of the femoral head, pathological fractures, bone pain, 'Erlenmeyer flask' deformity of the distal femora and 'moth-eaten' trabeculae. Hepatosplenomegaly is characteristic.

The third child has Lesch–Nyhan syndrome. It is an X-linked recessive condition which arises due to a deficiency in an enzyme critical for purine salvage. The purine salvage pathway is essential in many cells for DNA and RNA synthesis, as the capacity for de novo synthesis of purines can be insufficient. The deficient enzyme in Lesch–Nyhan syndrome is hypoxanthine guanine phosphoribosylpyrophosphate transferase (HGPRT). Without the salvaging of hypoxanthine and guanine by HGPRT, purines are shunted towards the excretion pathway. As these purines are degraded, large amounts of urate accumulate in the basal ganglia, kidney and circulation leading to hyperuricaemia, gouty arthritis and renal failure. Other manifestations include mental retardation, spastic cerebral palsy, self-mutilation and death often in the first decade. Orange crystals in diapers are an early sign. These are needle-shaped sodium urate crystals. Treatment with allopurinol is beneficial.

4. 1. **h. Haemangioma**. 2. **d. Osteochondroma**. 3. **c. Giant cell tumour**.
Vertical striations in a vertebral body on a plain radiograph are typical for haemangioma. This appearance has been described as 'jail-bar', 'honey-comb' and 'corduroy'. It occurs secondary to erosion of the horizontal trabeculae.

Osteochondromas typically have a cavity which is continuous with the medullary cavity of the origination. They can be sessile or pedunculated and may be investigated further with MRI scanning to assess the cartilage cap.

Giant cell tumour is most commonly found in the knee and distal radius. It is often eccentrically placed to the long axis of the bone. It is lytic, found in the metaphysis, stops short of the joint, thins the cortex and can expand into the surrounding soft tissues.

5. 1. **d. IgA**. 2. **k. Type IV hypersensitivity**. 3. **c. Complement factors**.
The first patient has selective IgA deficiency. She therefore has circulating antibodies to IgA. Fatal anaphylaxis may ensue if these patients are transfused with blood products, which frequently have serum containing IgA. It is therefore vital to ask about transfusion reactions when taking a history from an orthopaedic patient. Many patients with selective IgA deficiency are asymptomatic and are only diagnosed when they have an adverse transfusion reaction.

Metal allergy and sensitivity is becoming an increasingly recognized problem in orthopaedics, particularly with the renewed interest in metal-on-metal hip articulations. Skin allergy against metals is a well-recognized condition with nickel being the most common. It occurs in women who use cheap earrings or other jewellery made from high-nickel alloys. Some reports say that about 10% of the population suffers from this form of metal allergy. These patients suffer skin rash and eczema when in contact with objects containing high concentrations of nickel. This is an example of type IV hypersensitivity, where sensitized T lymphocytes encounter antigen and then release lymphokines, leading to macrophage activation. Whether metal allergy can cause implants, and in particular hip replacements, to fail is still a subject of much debate and research.

The third patient has disseminated gonococcal infection giving rise to gonococcal arthritis. Patients who have a complement factor deficiency of C5–C8 (membrane attack complex) are susceptible to Gram-negative bacteraemia, especially *Neisseria meningitidis*. Females are at particular risk of gonococcaemia during menstruation since sloughing of the endometrium allows access to the underlying blood supply and the necrotic tissue enhances growth of the bacteria.

6. 1. j. Aneurysmal bone cyst. 2. i. Tumoral calcinosis. 3. b. Melorheostosis.
Aneurysmal bone cysts usually occur in the metaphysis and tend to affect patients below the age of 20. They present with pain and swelling and can mimick a telangiectatic osteosarcoma. Radiographs show a typical 'bubbly' appearance with an expansile, lytic, septated lesion in the metaphysis. MRI or CT will show multiple fluid lines. The recommended treatment is aggressive curettage and grafting.

Tumoral calcinosis is a poorly understood condition characterized by extra-articular deposits of calcium typically around the hip and shoulder joints. It occurs more frequently in females and Afro-Caribbeans. The lesions are slow growing and rarely cause pain. Surgical excision is the treatment of choice for symptomatic deposits.

Melorheostosis is a connective tissue disorder characterized by thickening of cortices. Patients generally complain of joint pain, stiffness and deformity. The radiological appearance is one of wax dripping down the side of a candle.

7. 1. d. 'Alphabet soup' pattern. 2. a. 'Birbeck' granules. 3. h. 'Chicken wire' calcification.
Osteofibrous dysplasia is a rare, benign fibro-osseous lesion that occurs in children, almost exclusively confined to the anterior cortex of the tibia. The characteristic histological feature is of fibroblastic proliferation surrounding woven bone which gives an appearance of an 'alphabet soup' or 'Chinese letters'. This feature is also seen in fibrous dysplasia, but the key differentiating feature is osteoblastic rimming of the woven bone which is only seen in osteofibrous dysplasia.

Langerhans' cell histiocytosis (LCH) is a spectrum of diseases of the reticuloendothelial system that includes:

Eosinophilic granuloma (monostotic LCH)
Hand–Schüller–Christian disease (polyostotic LCH which can also include exophthalmus, diabetes insipidus and lytic skull lesions)
Letterer–Siwe disease (fatal form occurring in young patients)

Radiographs show a typically well-defined intramedullary lytic or 'punched-out' lesion in the diaphysis of long bones. The key histological feature is the Langerhans' cell which under electron microscopy has 'racquet-shaped' cytoplasmic inclusion bodies called 'Birbeck' granules.

Chondroblastoma is a benign chondrogenic lesion that occurs in young patients and is epiphyseal in location. The classic histological characteristics are chondroblasts arranged in a closely packed fashion with pericellular calcification that appears like 'chicken wire'.

8. 1. **j. Rifampicin**. 2. **g. Tetracyclines**. 3. **k. Trimethoprim**.
Rifampicin is an antitubercular drug. It blocks bacterial RNA synthesis and therefore transcription by inhibiting a DNA-dependent RNA polymerase. Its side effects include hepatitis and induction of cytochrome P450, which can decrease the efficacy of drugs given concomitantly, such as warfarin. Its most characteristic side effect is that it can make urine turn a red-orange colour.

The tetracylines are bacteriostatic drugs that block the elongation step in bacterial RNA translation. They prevent aminoacyl-tRNA from binding to the acceptor site on the 30S ribosomal subunit thus preventing a bacterial protein from being assembled. The most likely tetracycline that an orthopaedic surgeon is likely to use in his practice is doxycycline, which is the drug of choice for Lyme disease.

Trimethoprim prevents bacterial cell growth by inhibiting a key enzyme in folic acid synthesis: dihydrofolate reductase. This results in blocking the production of tetrahydrofolate which is required in purine and pyrimidine synthesis, which are in turn used for bacterial DNA and RNA synthesis.

9. 1. **f. *Peptostreptococcus***. 2. **l. *Streptococcus viridans***. 3. **g. *Borrelia burgdorferi***.
The most common organism infecting a joint replacement after a dental procedure is peptostreptococcus. Prophylactic antibiotics are not universally recommended to patients with joint replacements undergoing dental procedures.

There are numerous organisms which can be isolated after a 'fight bite'. From the choices available, E, F and N would all be reasonable answers for organisms found in human bite injuries. However, alpha-haemolytic streptococci are the most frequent isolates from human bite injuries, thus making *Streptococcus viridans* the best answer.

Lyme disease is important for the orthopaedic surgeon to recognize as it can present with acute, self-limiting joint effusions, in particular of the knee and shoulder. It is caused by the spirochete *Borrelia burdorferi* which is transmitted by the Ixodes tick. The classic presentation is erythema chronicum migrans, which is an expanding 'bulls-eye' red rash with central clearing. Bell's palsy is common, as are cardiac manifestations.

10. 1. **e. Multifocal osteomyelitis**. 2. **j. B, C**. 3. **d. Garre's sclerosing osteomyelitis**.
The first patient has a multifocal osteomyelitis. Many names have been used to describe this rare condition including chronic multifocal osteomyelitis and chronic recurrent multifocal osteomyelitis. It most commonly affects children who present with pain in the tibia, fibula, femur and clavicle. The natural history is self-limiting. A raised ESR is usually the only finding on the blood tests and cultures are frequently negative. The prognosis for these patients is good. In one study, 17 of 23 patients had complete resolution of the clinical findings, at an average of 5.6 years after diagnosis.

The second case is typical of a subacute osteomyelitis. The presentation is indolent and the diagnosis is usually made radiologically in a patient with a slowly progressing painful limp. The patient is systemically well and blood tests are normal. In some cases it may arise secondary to a partially treated acute osteomyelitis. The radiographic features described in this case are typical of a Brodie's abscess although the appearance can be difficult to differentiate from a Ewing's sarcoma. Once a malignancy has been ruled out, curettage and antibiotics form the mainstay of treatment.

Garre's sclerosing osteomyelitis is a rare form of osteomyelitis that involves the diaphyseal bones of adolescents. It is typified by a non-suppurative ossifying periostitis which may be caused by anaerobic organisms. Radiographs show a dense, progressive sclerosis. Malignancy must be ruled out by biopsy, and antibiotics are used in the treatment once the underlying cause has been addressed.

11. 1. m. Amputation. 2. g. Angiographic embolization. 3. o. I and K.
Having had two attempts at curettage without success, a ray amputation needs to be seriously considered here. Giant cell tumour in the hand is rare and we have treated such cases with amputation, achieving good patient satisfaction. Another option that can be used is to replace the metacarpal with a fibular strut graft attached to a Swanson's metacarpophalangeal joint replacement.

Resection of a solitary renal metastasis can be curative. These metastases however are extremely vascular. Many studies have now shown that preoperative embolization of feeder vessels is safe and effective in reducing blood loss at the time of excision of these tumours.

There is a wealth of evidence to now suggest that the best treatment for Ewing's sarcoma is neoadjuvant chemotherapy followed by wide excision and then maintenance chemotherapy. Due to the age and location of this boy's tumour, he will need endoprosthetic replacement in the form of a non-invasive growing distal femoral replacement. The initial results of non-invasive growers at our institution are very encouraging. We perform the lengthening every 4–6 weeks by a few millimetres using a magnet, in the outpatient setting.

12. 1. h. t (X:18). 2. a. pRB-1. 3. f. t (2:13).
Synovial sarcoma is the most common sarcoma found in the foot. It is a highly malignant lesion that arises proximal to joints but not within the joint. The chromosomal translocation t (X:18) is found in over 90% of cases. Despite wide excision, recurrence is common. The 10-year survival rate is 20%.

The second patient has had retinoblastoma and now has developed osteosarcoma. She is therefore homozygous for the retinoblastoma gene locus on chromosome 13. pRB-1 is a tumour suppressor gene and a mutation is found in 30% of osteosarcomas.

Rhabdomyosarcoma is the most common sarcoma in children and is associated with the t (2:13) translocation. Treatment includes chemotherapy, wide surgical resection and external beam irradiation.

13. 1. b. Systemic lupus erythematosus (SLE). 2. g. Gout. 3. j. CREST syndrome.
SLE is a chronic inflammatory disease which tends to affect women. Joint involvement is very common and includes the proximal interphalangeal (PIP), metacarpophalangeal (MCP) and knees. It is not as destructive as rheumatoid arthritis.

The punched-out periarticular lesions would suggest that this man has gout. His serum urate would be raised although this is not diagnostic. Monosodium urate crystals are found in the joint aspirate and demonstrating their presence is essential for diagnosis. They are thin, tapered and strongly negatively birefringent under polarized light.

Scleroderma can occur as systemic sclerosis or CREST syndrome. Systemic sclerosis is rapidly progressive and has early visceral involvement. CREST syndrome is what this lady has with: Calcinosis, Raynaud's phenomenon, Esophageal dysmotility, Sclerodactyly and Telangiectasia.

14. 1. h. Panner's disease. 2. f. Sever's disease. 3. c. Kohler's disease.
This question is an exercise in testing your recall with regard to the osteochondroses. You will just have to learn them! They arise at traction apophyses in children and may also be associated with trauma and inflammation.

15. 1. c. Warfarin. 2. e. Rivaroxaban. 3. f. Dabigatran.
Warfarin inhibits vitamin K epoxide. Factors II, VII, IX and X, which are vitamin K dependent, cannot therefore undergo post-translation modification and become active. Rifampicin induces the hepatic microsomal enzyme, cytochrome P450, which reduces the efficacy of warfarin.

Rivaroxaban is an orally active, direct factor Xa inhibitor. It is well absorbed from the gut and maximum inhibition of factor Xa occurs at 4 hours. It is dosed at once daily as its effect can last 8–12 hours. The attraction to using this drug for prophylaxis in orthopaedic patients is its oral bioavailability and once daily dosing regime.

Dabigatran is from the family of direct thrombin inhibitors. It has a number of important advantages over warfarin such as the lack of need for monitoring, a wide safety window and no reported major interactions with other drugs.

Selected references

Anderton JM. Orthopaedic problems in adult hypophosphatasia. *J Bone Joint Surg Br* 1979; **61**: 82–4.

Arnett FC, Edworthy SM, Bloch DA *et al.* The American Rheumatism Association 1987 revised criteria for the classification of rheumatoid arthritis. *Arthritis Rheum* 1988; **31**(3): 315–24.

Clark JCM, Dass CR, Choong PFM. A review of clinical and molecular prognostic factors in osteosarcoma. *J Cancer Res Clin Oncol* 2007; **134**(3): 281–97.

Damron TA, Beauchamp CP, Rougraff BT *et al.* Soft-tissue lumps and bumps. *Instr Course Lect* 2004; **53**: 625–37.

Desai SS, Jambhekar N, Agarwal M, Puri A, Merchant N. Adamantinoma of tibia: a study of 12 cases. *J Surg Oncol* 2006; **93**: 429–33.

DiCaprio MR, Enneking WF. Fibrous dysplasia: pathophysiology, evaluation, and treatment. *J Bone Joint Surg Am* 2005; **87**: 1848–64.

Enneking WF, Spannier SS, Goodman MA. A system for the surgical staging of musculoskeletal sarcoma. *Clin Orthop Relat Res* 1980; **153**: 106–20.

Goldstein EJ, Citron DM, Wield B *et al.* Bacteriology of human and animal bite wounds. *J Clin Microbiol* 1978; **8**(6): 667–72.

Helms CA. *Fundamentals of Skeletal Radiology*, 2nd edn. Philadelphia, WB Saunders, 1994.

Huber AM, Lam PY, Duffy CM *et al.* Chronic recurrent multifocal osteomyelitis: clinical outcomes after more than five years of follow-up. *J Pediatr* 2002; **141**: 198–203.

Levinson W, Jawetz E. *Medical Microbiology and Immunology*, 5th edn. Maidenhead, Appleton and Lange, 1998.

Mackenzie WG, Morton KS. Eosinophilic granuloma of bone. *Can J Surg* 1988; **31**(4): 264–7.

Martinez S. Tumoral calcinosis: 12 years later. *Semin Musculoskelet Radiol* 2002; **6**(4): 331–9. Review.

Menendez LR. (ed.) *Orthopaedic Knowledge Update: Musculoskeletal Tumors.* Rosemont, IL, American Academy of Orthopaedic Surgeons. 2002; pp. 305–12.

Miller MD. *Review of Orthopaedics*, 5th edn. Philadelphia, Elsevier, 2008.

Nyhan WL. The recognition of Lesch-Nyhan syndrome as an inborn error of purine metabolism. *J Inherit Metab Dis* 1997; **20**(2): 171–8.

Pastores GM, Patel MJ, Firooznia H. Bone and joint complications related to Gaucher's disease. *Curr Rheumatol Rep* 2000; **2**: 175–80.

Pitcher JD Jr, Weber KL. Benign fibrous and histiocytic lesions. In: Schwartz HS, ed. *Orthopaedic Knowledge Update: Musculoskeletal Tumors* 2. Rosemont, IL, American Academy of Orthopaedic Surgeons. 2007; 121–32.

Prabhu VC, Bilsky MH, Jambhekar K *et al.* Results of preoperative embolization for metastatic spinal neoplasms. *J Neurosurg* 2003; **98**: 156–64.

Robin NH, Shprintzen RJ. Defining the clinical spectrum of deletion 22q11.2. *J Pediatr* 2005; **147**(1): 90–6.

Schulman S, Kearon C, Kakkar AK *et al.* Dabigatran versus warfarin in the treatment of acute venous thromboembolism. *N Engl J Med* 2009; **361**(24): 2342–52.

Simon MA, Springfield DS. (eds.) *Surgery of Bone and Soft-Tissue Tumors*. Philadelphia, PA, Lippincott-Raven. 1998; 190–1.

Suma R, Vinay C, Shashikanth MC, Subba Reddy VV Garre's sclerosing osteomyelitis. *J Indian Soc Pedod Prev Dent* 2007; **25** Suppl: S30–3.

Van der Linden S, Valkenburg HA, Cats A. Evaluation of diagnostic criteria for ankylosing spondylitis. A proposal for modification of the New York criteria. *Arthritis Rheum* 1987; **27**(4): 361–8.

Paediatric orthopaedics: Questions

Russell Hawkins and Deborah M. Eastwood

MCQs

1. **Which of the following is the most sensitive clinical sign for detection of developmental dysplasia of the hip (DDH) in a baby aged 6 months?**
   a. Galeazzi test.
   b. Asymmetric skin folds in the thighs.
   c. Limited hip abduction in flexion.
   d. Ortolani's test.
   e. Barlow's test.

2. **On an anteroposterior (AP) radiograph, which of the following defines a B/C border hip according to Herring's modified classification of Perthes disease?**
   a. A very narrow lateral pillar which is <50% of the original height.
   b. A lateral pillar with very little ossification with at least 50% of the original height.
   c. A lateral pillar with increased ossification with at least 50% of the original height.
   d. A lateral pillar with exactly 50% of the original height that is higher than the central pillar.
   e. Gage's sign.

3. **When treating slipped upper femoral epiphysis (SUFE), which of the following might be the sole indication for subcapital osteotomy?**
   a. Metaphyseal blanch sign.
   b. Southwick angle >60°.
   c. Avascular necrosis (AVN).
   d. Femoral retroversion.
   e. Endocrinopathy.

4. **When investigating for the presence of femoroacetabular impingement (FAI), which of the following radiographic views is most likely to identify a cam lesion?**
   a. Cross table lateral.
   b. False profile.
   c. Frog lateral.
   d. Billings lateral.
   e. Dunn lateral.

Postgraduate Orthopaedics, ed. Kesavan Sri-Ram. Published by Cambridge University Press.
© Cambridge University Press 2012.

5. **Which of the following is the best predictor of avascular necrosis (AVN) following hip fracture in children?**
   a. Fracture type and patient age.
   b. Open anatomical reduction and rigid internal fixation.
   c. Surgery within 36 hours and capsular decompression.
   d. Initial displacement and associated injuries.
   e. Hospital type and grade of surgeon.

6. **A supracondylar fracture of the distal humerus with posterolateral displacement should be reduced by performing reduction manoeuvres in the following order?**
   a. Valgus – Flexion – Pronation.
   b. Varus – Extension – Supination.
   c. Valgus – Extension – Pronation.
   d. Traction – Pronation – Flexion.
   e. Varus – Extension – Pronation.

7. **Following clubfoot surgery, which of the following is the commonest residual deformity?**
   a. Forefoot adduction.
   b. Internal tibial torsion.
   c. Forefoot supination.
   d. Equinus.
   e. Hindfoot varus.

8. **Which of the following is not a typical deformity/gait disturbance seen in cerebral palsy?**
   a. Toe walking.
   b. Wide-based gait.
   c. Hip adduction.
   d. Wrist flexion.
   e. Forearm supination.

9. **Which of the following is not a component of Kocher's criteria when diagnosing septic arthritis of the hip?**
   a. Non-weight-bearing on the affected side.
   b. Erythrocyte sedimentation rate (ESR) greater than 40 mm/hr.
   c. Fever.
   d. White blood cell (WBC) count of $>12\,000\,mm^3$.
   e. C-reactive protein (CRP) >20.

10. **Which of the following is not a characteristic abnormality in fibular hemimelia?**
    a. Genu valgum.
    b. Coxa vara.
    c. Posteromedial tibial bowing.
    d. Flattened tibial spine.
    e. Hypoplastic lateral femoral condyle.

11. **Using the 'rule of thumb', to the nearest half centimetre what is the combined remaining growth from the distal femoral and proximal tibial physes in a 12-year-old girl with a bone age matched to her chronological age.**
    a. 2.0 cm.
    b. 2.5 cm.
    c. 3.0 cm.
    d. 3.5 cm.
    e. 4.0 cm.

12. **After the age of 4, the proximal femoral epiphysis receives its predominant blood supply via an increased contribution from which of the following?**
    a. Ligamentum teres.
    b. Metaphyseal vessels.
    c. Lateral circumflex vessels.
    d. Medial circumflex vessels.
    e. Anterosuperior branches.

13. **Which of the following has the greatest specificity for non-accidental injury (NAI)?**
    a. Metaphyseal corner fractures.
    b. Skull fractures.
    c. Vertebral fractures.
    d. Isolated rib fractures.
    e. Scapular fractures.

14. **Which is the least important risk factor associated with developmental dysplasia of the hip?**
    a. Female sex.
    b. Breech position.
    c. Positive family history.
    d. Gestational diabetes.
    e. First born child.

15. **Which of the following is not associated with rhabdomyosarcoma?**
    a. High malignancy.
    b. myoD1 protein.
    c. Most commonly a tumour of the head and neck.
    d. Chemoresistance.
    e. Radiosensitivity.

16. **In relation to Tillaux fractures, in which order does the distal tibial physis close?**
    a. Central – medial – lateral; anterior – posterior.
    b. Central – lateral – medial; anterior – posterior.
    c. Central – medial – lateral; posterior – anterior.
    d. Central – lateral – medial; posterior – anterior.
    e. Medial – central – lateral; posterior – anterior.

17. In Risser staging, an iliac apophysis showing 75% ossification represents which of the following?
    a. Risser 1.
    b. Risser 2.
    c. Risser 3.
    d. Risser 4.
    e. Risser 5.

18. Which zone of the physis is predominantly affected by fibroblast growth factors?
    a. Resting.
    b. Proliferative.
    c. Hypertrophic.
    d. Calcification.
    e. Primary spongiosa.

19. Which of the following is not a feature of achondroplasia?
    a. Long fibula.
    b. Normal sitting height.
    c. Short pedicles.
    d. Coxa vara.
    e. Radial head subluxation.

20. Which of the following is not associated with spina bifida/neural tube defects?
    a. Increased frequency of lower limb fractures.
    b. Increased maternal serum/amniotic fluid alpha-fetoprotein levels.
    c. Hyperhomocysteinaemia.
    d. Budd–Chiari syndrome.
    e. Syringomyelia.

21. Regarding endotracheal intubation in paediatric trauma, which of the following is not a consideration of airway management in children compared to adults?
    a. Large occiput.
    b. Large tongue.
    c. Anterior larynx.
    d. Greater accumulation of secretions.
    e. More difficult cord visualization in neutral position.

22. Which of the following procedures is appropriate in the setting of an increased TT-TG (tibial tuberosity–centre of trochlear groove) offset >15 mm in the treatment of chronic patellofemoral instability?
    a. Elmslie–Trillat procedure.
    b. Distalizing tibial tubercle transfer.
    c. Trochleoplasty.
    d. Lateral release.
    e. Medial patellofemoral ligament (MPFL) reconstruction.

23. Regarding embryological limb bud formation, which of the following is responsible for longitudinal growth of the limb?
    a. Sonic hedgehog genes.
    b. Apoptosis.

    c. Homeobox genes.

    d. Noggin.

    e. Zone of proliferating activity.

24. **Which of the following statements is incorrect: Ultrasound examination is an imperfect screening tool in the diagnosis of developmental dysplasia of the hip (DDH) because?**

    a. DDH has a known incidence.

    b. There is an accepted and effective treatment.

    c. Examination is acceptable to the carers.

    d. The effect of early treatment is unknown.

    e. Non-invasive treatment causes avascular necrosis (AVN).

25. **Regarding tarsal coalition, which of the following is not associated with a calcaneonavicular bar?**

    a. Autosomal dominance.

    b. Anteater sign.

    c. Posterior facet subtalar arthrosis.

    d. Presentation at 12–16 years.

    e. 20% incidence of multiple coalitions.

26. **Regarding congenital hand anomalies, which of the following is characterized by fixed ulnar bowing of a digit?**

    a. Brachysyndactyly.

    b. Camptodactyly.

    c. Clinodactyly.

    d. Acrosyndactyly.

    e. Symphalangism.

27. **Which is the most common site of pelvic apophyseal avulsion fractures?**

    a. Lesser trochanter.

    b. Anterior superior iliac spine (ASIS).

    c. Anterior inferior iliac spine (AIIS).

    d. Pubic tubercle.

    e. Ischial tuberosity.

28. **On a pelvic radiograph, which line passes through the inferior teardrop and joins the superolateral and inferomedial aspects of the bony socket?**

    a. Hilgenreiner's.

    b. Perkin's.

    c. Shenton's.

    d. Wiberg's.

    e. Sharp's

29. **Regarding obstetric brachial plexus injuries, which of the following is not typically associated with Erb's palsy?**

    a. Anterior shoulder dislocation.

    b. Shoulder adduction.

   c. Elbow extension.

   d. Increased likelihood of skin infections.

   e. Forearm pronation.

30. **According to Rubin's classification of skeletal dysplasias, where would you place 'Trevor's disease'?**

   a. Epiphyseal hyperplasia

   b. Physeal hypoplasia.

   c. Metaphyseal hypoplasia.

   d. Metaphyseal hyperplasia.

   e. Diaphyseal hyperplasia.

EMQs

1. **Inherited conditions**
   a. Fibroblast growth factor receptor 3 (FGFR3)
   b. X-linked recessive
   c. PEX
   d. Type I collagen
   e. Sulphate transporter
   f. Fibrillin
   g. Core binding factor alpha-1 (CBFA1)
   h. Type II collagen
   i. Cartilage oligomeric matrix protein (COMP)
   j. Type X collagen

Which of the options above is best described in each of the following statements? Each option may be used once, more than once or not at all.
   1. Associated with an X-linked dominant condition.
   2. Associated with a condition characterized by absent clavicles.
   3. Associated with a condition presenting with Gower's sign.

2. **Classifications in paediatric orthopaedics**
   a. Achtermann and Kalamchi
   b. Aiken
   c. Crowe
   d. King and Moe
   e. Graf
   f. Harcke
   g. Dimeglio
   h. Ratliff
   i. Wassel
   j. Kalamchi and MacEwen

Which of the options above is best described in each of the following statements? Each option may be used once, more than once or not at all.
   1. A classification of post-traumatic avascular necrosis.
   2. A dynamic classification of developmental dysplasia of the hip (DDH) using ultrasound.
   3. A classification of a post-axial limb deficiency.

3. **Congenital deformities**
   a. Phocomelia
   b. Radial club hand
   c. TAR syndrome
   d. VACTERL syndrome
   e. Sprengel's shoulder
   f. Sacral agenesis
   g. Fibular hemimelia

h. Clinodactyly
i. Polydactyly
j. Radial head dislocation

Which of the options above is best described in each of the following statements? Each option may be used once, more than once or not at all.
1. A condition classically associated with maternal diabetes.
2. A condition associated with the omovertebral bone.
3. A condition recognizable on antenatal ultrasound as a marker for Down syndrome (and other chromosomal anomalies).

4. **Paediatric fractures**
  a. Salter–Harris I
  b. Greenstick
  c. Salter–Harris II
  d. Torus
  e. Salter–Harris III
  f. Avulsion
  g. Salter–Harris IV
  h. Non-accidental injury
  i. Salter–Harris VI
  j. Salter–Harris V

Which of the options above is best described in each of the following statements? Each option may be used once, more than once or not at all.
1. Injury to the perichondral ring.
2. A type of acetabular injury with the worst outcome.
3. Supination-inversion injury to the medial malleolus.

5. **Metabolic bone disease**
  a. Vitamin D-dependent rickets
  b. Hypophosphatasia
  c. Albright's syndrome
  d. Hypothyroidism
  e. Vitamin D-resistant rickets
  f. Milk-alkali syndrome
  g. Vitamin D-deficiency rickets
  h. Renal osteodystrophy
  i. Osteopetrosis
  j. Osteomalacia

Which of the options above is best described in each of the following statements? Each option may be used once, more than once or not at all.
1. A condition that can cause anaemia.
2. A condition giving the appearances of bilateral Perthes disease.
3. The commonest bone mineralization defect.

6. Bone tumours and tumour-like conditions
   a. Osteoid osteoma
   b. Ewing's sarcoma
   c. Rhabdomyosarcoma
   d. Leukaemia
   e. Osteosarcoma
   f. Fibrous dysplasia
   g. Non-ossifying fibroma
   h. Adamantinoma
   i. Neuroblastoma
   j. Langerhans' cell histiocytosis

Which of the options above is best described in each of the following statements? Each option may be used once, more than once or not at all.
   1. A condition associated with genetic translocation t (11:22).
   2. When associated with soft tissue tumours is termed Mazabraud's syndrome.
   3. Has a lesion typically <2 cm diameter.

7. Neuromuscular conditions
   a. Cerebral palsy
   b. Duchenne's muscular dystrophy
   c. Charcot–Marie–Tooth disease
   d. Friedreich's ataxia
   e. Arthrogryposis
   f. Myelodysplasia
   g. Spinal muscular atrophy
   h. Dejerine–Sottas disease
   i. Poliomyelitis
   j. Myaesthenia gravis

Which of the options above is best described in each of the following statements? Each option may be used once, more than once or not at all.
   1. A contraindication to the use of botulinum toxin.
   2. Associated with genetic defect of PMP22.
   3. A condition caused by mitochondrial dysfunction.

8. Causative pathogens
   a. *Salmonella*
   b. Herpes simplex virus
   c. *Streptococcus viridans*
   d. Group B streptococci
   e. *Staphylococcus aureus*
   f. *Streptococcus pneumoniae*
   g. *Neisseria gonorrhoeae*
   h. *Haemophilus influenzae*
   i. *Enterobacter*
   j. *Mycobacterium tuberculosis*

Which of the options above is best described in each of the following statements? Each
option may be used once, more than once or not at all.
1. Commonest pathogen causing bone and joint infections in the neonate.
2. Commonest pathogen causing bone and joint infections in a 5-year-old.
3. Commonest pathogen causing bone and joint infections in a patient with sickle
   cell disease.

9. **Foot disorders**
   a. Congenital vertical talus
   b. Skewfoot
   c. Habitual toe walking
   d. Congenital talipes equinovarus (CTEV)
   e. Metatarsus adductus
   f. Tarsal coalition
   g. Pes planovalgus
   h. Claw foot
   i. Ball and socket ankle
   j. Pes cavovarus

Which of the options above is best described in each of the following statements? Each
option may be used once, more than once or not at all.
1. Requires calcaneal osteotomy if the Coleman block test does not correct hindfoot
   deformity.
2. Fixed equinus hindfoot with irreducible dorsal dislocation of navicular.
3. A valgus hindfoot with an adducted forefoot.

10. **Spinal disorders**
    a. Scheuermann's disease
    b. Osteoblastoma
    c. Myelodysplasia
    d. Adolescent idiopathic scoliosis
    e. Spondylolysis
    f. Hemivertebrae
    g. Syringomyelia
    h. Flat back syndrome
    i. Discitis
    j. Diastomatomyelia

Which of the options above is best described in each of the following statements? Each
option may be used once, more than once or not at all.
1. Seen on oblique views of the lumbar spine.
2. A complication of scoliosis surgery.
3. A form of juvenile osteochondritis.

11. **Radiological signs**
    a. Fallen fragment
    b. Gage's

c. Metaphyseal blanch
d. Sunray spicules
e. Rugger jersey
f. Erlenmeyer flask
g. Looser's zones
h. Codman's triangle
i. Sagging rope
j. Bone within a bone

Which of the options above is best described in each of the following statements? Each option may be used once, more than once or not at all.
1. Condition involving carbonic anhydrase deficiency.
2. Condition associated with avascular necrosis (AVN) and abnormal growth of the femoral epiphysis.
3. Condition predominantly seen in the proximal humerus.

12. **Hip disorders**
    a. Avascular necrosis (AVN)
    b. Septic arthritis
    c. Slipped upper femoral epiphysis (SUFE)
    d. Femoroacetabular impingement
    e. Developmental dysplasia of the hip (DDH)
    f. Snapping fascia lata
    g. Perthes disease
    h. Coxa vara
    i. Epiphysiolysis
    j. Transient synovitis

Which of the options above is best described in each of the following statements? Each option may be used once, more than once or not at all.
1. May be associated with a positive Ober test.
2. A condition where damage occurs at the chondrolabral junction.
3. May be diagnosed with Trethowan's sign.

13. **Pelvic osteotomies**
    a. Ganz
    b. Pemberton
    c. Greenfield
    d. Salter
    e. Sutherland
    f. Tonnis
    g. Steel
    h. Chiari
    i. Triple
    j. Shelf

Which of the options above is best described in each of the following statements? Each option may be used once, more than once or not at all.

1. An osteotomy which hinges on the triradiate cartilage.
2. A medial displacement salvage osteotomy to improve lateral cover.
3. Also known as the 'Bernese' osteotomy.

14. **Numeric values**
   a. 1
   b. 2
   c. 3
   d. 4
   e. 5
   f. 6
   g. 7
   h. 8
   i. 9
   j. 10

Which of the options above is best described in each of the following statements? Each option may be used once, more than once or not at all.

1. The expected age of a patient whose trochlear ossification centre is visible on plain radiographs of the elbow.
2. The cervical nerve root value affected in Klumpke's obstetric palsy.
3. The average percentage recurrence rate following excision of a malignant musculoskeletal tumour with a wide margin.

15. **Apophyseal conditions and associated traction injuries**
   a. Medial epicondyle
   b. Inferior patellar
   c. Calcaneum
   d. Ischial tuberosity
   e. Anterior superior iliac spine (ASIS)
   f. Tibial tubercle
   g. Greater trochanter
   h. Iliac crest
   i. Lesser trochanter
   j. Anterior inferior iliac spine (AIIS)

Which of the options above is best described in each of the following statements? Each option may be used once, more than once or not at all.

1. The affected area in Sinding-Larsen–Johansson syndrome.
2. Site of potential apophyseal avulsion during tennis serves.
3. Apophysis appearing at age 5 years.

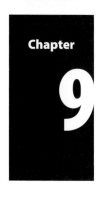

Paediatric orthopaedics: Answers

Russell Hawkins and Deborah M. Eastwood

MCQs

1. c. Limited hip abduction in flexion.
Less than 60° of abduction at 90° of hip flexion is the most sensitive clinical test especially in the older child (>3 months) when the Barlow and Ortolani tests become less reliable. Neither the Barlow nor the Ortolani test will detect an irreducible dislocated hip. The Galeazzi test may reveal unilateral shortening but this may be attributable to causes other than DDH (for example congenital coxa vara). False-negative results are seen in cases of bilateral DDH (20% of DDH cases). Asymmetric skin folds are non-specific and seen in 25% of normal babies.

2. b. A lateral pillar with very little ossification with at least 50% of the original height.
The original Herring classification (A,B,C) using the lateral pillar height was modified to define more accurately those hips at the borders of those groups. The definition of group A remained a hip with no density changes in the lateral pillar and no loss of the height of the lateral pillar. Group B describes hips with a lateral pillar of >50% of the original height, a width of more than a few millimetres, and substantial ossification. Group C is defined as hips with collapse of the lateral pillar beyond 50% of the original height. The B/C border hip is now defined as either (1) a very narrow lateral pillar (2 to 3 mm wide) that is >50% of the original height; or (2) a lateral pillar with very little ossification but with at least 50% of the original height or (3) a lateral pillar with exactly 50% of the original height that is depressed relative to the central pillar.

3. b. Southwick angle >60°.
The most frequently quoted and used Southwick angle is measured on a frog lateral view of both hips and defined as the difference in the head-shaft angles following SUFE. (An anteroposterior (AP) angle has also been reported but is used less commonly.) The head-shaft angle is determined by the intersection of a line perpendicular to the axis between the anterior and posterior tips of the epiphysis at the physis and a line along the anatomical axis of the femur. The value for the normal side is then subtracted from that of the slipped side and the angle calculated determines the severity. Mild is <30°, moderate is 30–60° and severe is >60°. 12° is the normal control value and can be used in the case of bilateral involvement. There is some controversy in the literature as to whether 50° or 60° is the 'cut-off' between moderate and severe – this probably relates to whether or not the 'normal' side has in fact been subtracted from the value for the abnormal side. The term

Postgraduate Orthopaedics, ed. Kesavan Sri-Ram. Published by Cambridge University Press.
© Cambridge University Press 2011.

'slip angle' is commonly used but is rarely defined: it usually refers to the Southwick angle (with or without subtraction of the normal side). Severe slips treated with pinning *in situ* show poorer results than mild and moderate slips. The metaphyseal blanch sign is a radiographic sign of SUFE seen on the AP pelvic radiograph. It can be seen even with minor slips. Recent publications suggest that AVN complicates 20% of acute, severe unstable slips. AVN is also a complication of subcapital osteotomy. It is not an indication for such an osteotomy. Femoral retroversion puts stress across the physis and is a mechanical factor associated with development of a SUFE. Endocrinopathy is a potential cause of SUFE and may guide the surgeon towards prophylactic pinning of the unaffected hip.

4. e. **Dunn lateral.**
Although most of these views can be used to identify cam lesions, the Dunn lateral view shows subtle increased prominence at the anterolateral head–neck junction, loss of the head–neck offset and increased radial curvature. It is taken with the patient supine with the hip flexed to either 45° or 90° with 20° of abduction and neutral or slight internal rotation. Cam lesions may occur secondary to congenital or acquired dysplasia such as incomplete remodelling following Perthes disease or slipped upper femoral epiphysis (SUFE).

5. a. **Fracture type and patient age.**
Paediatric hip trauma is uncommon (<1% of all paediatric fractures) and is associated with poor outcomes if complicated by AVN (or malunion). Because of its rarity, identifying the best method of treatment and those factors which truly predict AVN has been difficult to prove scientifically. Although the factors mentioned in this question may be associated with AVN, a meta-analysis of 360 cases shows only patient age and fracture type to be predictive of AVN. The older patient has less potential for revascularization and remodelling of the proximal femur and the more proximal intracapsular fractures are more sensitive to vascular disruption. Fractures are classified according to Delbet and Colonna; type I is transphyseal suffixed A if an associated dislocation is present and suffixed B if no dislocation. Type 2 is transcervical, type 3 cervico-trochanteric and type 4 intertrochanteric. Types 1–3 are intracapsular with type 1A carrying the highest risk of AVN at almost 100%. Type IV is extracapsular with the lowest risk of AVN.

6. b. **Varus – Extension – Supination.**
All supracondylar fractures should be reduced by correcting the coronal plane deformity first, followed by the sagittal plane and lastly the axial plane. The exact manoeuvres are determined by the direction of displacement and the location of the periosteal hinge. The more common posteromedial fractures have an intact medial periosteal hinge which aids fracture reduction when the forearm is pronated. The same manoeuvre performed for the less common posterolateral fracture will displace the distal fragment further owing to the lateral periosteal hinge and supination is therefore required to aid fracture reduction.

7. a. **Forefoot adduction.**
Forefoot adduction is the commonest residual (as distinct from recurrent) deformity in the treated clubfoot and results either from residual talonavicular subluxation or residual metatarsus varus. Radiographs show a short medial column and longer lateral column. The typical 'bean-shaped' foot may also be a product of an associated forefoot supination which is the second commonest residual deformity. Treatment may involve medial column

lengthening and lateral column shortening osteotomies in the absence of other contributing factors. When evaluating forefoot deformity, it is essential that the hindfoot is examined to ensure that hindfoot deformity is not giving the false impression of a forefoot problem. Residual forefoot adduction is much less of a problem following Ponseti treatment of the congenital talipes equinovarus (CTEV) deformity.

8. e. **Forearm supination.**
The typical hip deformities are flexion, adduction and internal rotation with this latter secondary to excessive femoral anteversion. Collectively, these contribute to a scissoring gait. The 'windswept deformity' may occur particularly in non-ambulatory patients where one hip is abducted and the other adducted. Typically, the knee is flexed. The common foot abnormalities are secondary to the tendency to toe walk and they include equinovalgus and equinovarus deformities. The upper limb tends to be affected by flexion of the elbow, wrist and fingers with or without the 'thumb in palm' deformity. Swan-necking of the fingers is also seen commonly. The forearm is usually pronated. The spine may demonstrate an increased lumbar lordosis, scoliosis or a kyphosis: often dependent on the predominant muscle tone (low or high). A 'wide-based gait' is seen in ataxic cerebral palsy.

9. e. **C-reactive protein (CRP) >20.**
Due to the rapid chondrolytic effect of pus within the joint, pyogenic septic arthritis of the hip in children represents a surgical emergency. It can be difficult to distinguish a septic hip from other causes of hip pain in children. In such cases, whilst clinical suspicion remains of paramount importance, Kocher's diagnostic algorithm is a useful tool. The four diagnostic criteria are non-weight-bearing, ESR >40, WBC >12 and fever. The predicted risk of a septic arthritis varies with the number of positive criteria. The algorithm has been tested retrospectively and prospectively. In the prospective validation study the probabilities were lower:

Number of criteria met	Chance of septic arthritis (original study)	Chance of septic arthritis (validation study)
1	3%	9.5%
2	40%	35%
3	93%	73%
4	99.6%	93%

10. c. **Posteromedial tibial bowing.**
Fibular hemimelia is a postaxial deficiency or dysplasia in which there is aplasia or variable hypoplasia of the fibula. There are a number of associated features comprising from distal to proximal: absent lateral rays and/or tarsal bones, tarsal coalition, ball and socket ankle, valgus ankle, anteromedial tibial bowing, flattened tibial spine, absent anterior cruciate ligament (ACL), genu valgum, hypoplastic lateral femoral condyle, lateral patellar subluxation, femoral hypoplasia, coxa vara and possibly a true proximal femoral focal deficiency (PFFD). Congenital posteromedial bowing of the infantile tibia is considered 'benign' in that the deformity improves with growth. However, there is often a significant residual leg length discrepancy.

11. c. **3.0 cm.**
Epiphysiodesis of the longer limb is used to treat predicted leg length discrepancies of 2–5 cm. The 'rule of thumb' serves as an estimate of remaining growth and therefore guides the surgeon when to perform epiphysiodesis. Lower limb growth occurs from four main physes: most growth occurs around the knee with the greatest contribution from the distal femoral physis at 10 mm per year. The proximal tibial physis contributes a further 6 mm per year with lesser contributions from the proximal femoral and the distal tibial physes (3–4 mm each). Physes are expected to close at approximately age 14 in girls (or 18 months after menarche) and age 16 in boys. Therefore, in this example, physeal closure is expected after 2 years giving a total of 32 mm $[(10 \times 2) + (6 \times 2)]$. However, the rule of thumb must be used with caution as bone age and the non-linear growth pattern of bones needs to be taken into account.

Aguilar *et al* have devised and validated a multiplier method for predicting growth and limb length discrepancy which may be more accurate but a little more time consuming and difficult to calculate.

12. d. **Medial circumflex vessels.**
The blood supply to the proximal femoral epiphysis is reported to change with age. Until age 4, the supply to the femoral head is derived equally from medial and lateral circumflex vessels as well as the ligamentum teres. The physis acts as a mechanical barrier with virtually no traversing metaphyseal vessels reaching the epiphysis. After age 4, supply from the ligamentum teres diminishes and the distribution of supply from the circumflex vessels changes; the lateral circumflex system supplies predominantly the metaphysis whilst the medial circumflex system becomes the predominant supply to the proximal femoral epiphysis via its posterosuperior branch. After age 10 years, supply by the ligamentum teres diminishes further and the femoral epiphysis relies upon the end arterial supply of the retinacular vessels. With the closure of the physis at skeletal maturity, anastamoses develop between the vessels of the ligamentum teres, epiphyseal and metaphyseal systems and there is less reliance on end arteries.

13. d. **Isolated rib fractures.**
The high incidence of fractures in NAI means that one-third of cases are eventually reviewed by an orthopaedic surgeon. Injury patterns vary with age and mobility of the child and an injury out of keeping with the child's developmental stage or where the mechanism does not fit should raise suspicion. No fracture is pathognomonic and the diagnosis is made on the basis of all the information available from the history, examination and investigation findings. However, certain fractures and patterns of injuries are associated with NAI. Isolated or multiple rib fractures are the most specific. Other associated fractures include those of the scapular, lateral clavicle, vertebrae and complex skull fractures (not linear fractures). Transphyseal fractures through the proximal femoral physis are commonly due to NAI in the non-ambulatory child. The pattern of injury is also important – soft tissue injuries accompanying fractures such as bruises, bites or burns are characteristic of NAI as are multiple fractures at different stages of healing and metaphyseal corner or bucket handle fractures.

14. d. **Gestational diabetes.**
The two most important risk factors for developmental dysplasia of the hip are a positive family history and breech position. The other important risk factors are first

born children and female sex. Gestational diabetes is not particularly associated with developmental dysplasia of the hip.

15. d. Chemoresistance.
Rhabdomyosarcoma is the commonest soft tissue sarcoma in children particularly under age 5. It is a highly malignant tumour formed from muscle cell progenitors. It can occur in regions with little skeletal muscle and most commonly presents as a tumour of the head and neck (40%) with a lower incidence in the extremities (20%). It is associated with persistence of the embryonal protein myoD1 that usually vanishes when normal muscle matures and becomes innervated. Histologically, the characteristic findings are spindle cells, giant cells and racquet cells. The rhabdomyoblasts are recognizable by their cross striations. These tumours are difficult to treat surgically but are both chemo- and radiosensitive. Patients commonly receive neoadjuvant chemotherapy followed by wide local excision and post-operative radiotherapy.

16. c. Central – medial – lateral; posterior – anterior.
A Tillaux fracture is a Salter–Harris III avulsion injury of the anterolateral distal tibial physis by the anterior tibiofibular ligament (ATFL). It occurs following a low energy external rotation injury mechanism between the ages of 11 and 15 more commonly in girls and during sporting activities. It is the sequence of physeal closure at the distal tibia which accounts for this pattern of injury. Physeal closure begins with the central third, followed by the medial third and lastly the lateral third. Closure also occurs in a posterior to anterior direction and therefore, with injury, the strong ATFL avulses the relatively weak anterolateral portion of the epiphysis. The fragment is usually displaced anterolaterally and there may be associated diastasis. The Tillaux fragment should be fixed if displacement is >2 mm.

17. c. Risser 3.
Risser staging 1–5 depends on the amount of ossification of the iliac apophysis visible on the anteroposterior (AP) radiograph. Ossification begins anterolaterally and proceeds posteromedially. The first 25% equates to Risser 1 and grade 4 equates to 100% ossification. Grade 5 is signified by fusion of the apophysis. The relevance of Risser staging is in predicting the progression of scoliotic curves. Small curves and greater skeletal maturity according to the Risser stage predicts a smaller likelihood of curve progression compared to larger curves and skeletal immaturity.

18. b. Proliferative.
Fibroblast growth factors (FGFs) affect the growth of long bones through stimulation of the proliferative zone. In achondroplasia, a defective FGF receptor gene (FGFR3) is responsible for the characteristic limb shortening.

19. d. Coxa vara.
Achondroplasia is a type of rhizomelic dwarfism caused by an autosomal dominant genetic defect in the FGFR3 gene that is responsible for long bone growth. Therefore, individuals may have a normal sitting height with a reduced standing height. Progressively short pedicles in the distal spine predispose the child to problems with spinal stenosis. There is often an excessive lumbar lordosis and a junctional kyphosis in the non-ambulant child.

Achondroplasia is associated with coxa valga and genu varum with a disproportionately long fibula whereas spondyloepiphyseal dysplasia congenita is associated with the opposite deformities of coxa vara and genu valgum. Other features of achondroplasia comprise frontal bossing, trident hands, radial bowing, radial head subluxation, a champagne glass pelvis, inverted V-shaped distal femoral physes and tibial bowing.

20. d. **Budd–Chiari syndrome.**
Neural tube defects (NTDs) are a spectrum of disorders caused by failure of the posterior neural elements to fuse at around 3–4 weeks' gestation. The causes are multifactorial although a raised level of homocysteine, a consequence of folate deficiency, is strongly implicated. NTDs are either open or closed. Open lesions usually involve the entire central nervous system (CNS) with leakage of cerebrospinal fluid (CSF) and result from failure of primary neurulation. Closed lesions are usually localized to the spine and result from failure of secondary neurulation. Closed types are covered by an epithelial layer and neural elements are therefore not exposed. However, any overlying skin may be dysplastic and cutaneous stigamata such as a pit or a hairy patch may be noticeable. The effects of NTDs depend on their location and severity although paralysis (flaccid and/or spastic) and bowel and bladder incontinence are characteristic. A type II Arnold–Chiari malformation is the commonest associated condition: downwards displacement of the cerebellar tonsils through the foramen magnum which can lead to hydrocephalus and mental retardation. Budd–Chiari syndrome is occlusion of the hepatic veins and is unrelated to NTDs.

21. e. **More difficult cord visualization in neutral position.**
When providing airway management to the paediatric trauma patient, the anatomical differences between children and adults must be considered. A relatively large occiput naturally flexes the C-spine causing buckling of the pharynx. A neutral position with the midface parallel to the spinal board is recommended. As the larynx is more anterior and cephalad, this position also improves visualization of the cords although a larger tongue and tonsils may interfere with this. The larynx is also funnel shaped allowing greater accumulation of secretions. A shorter trachea means a greater risk of right main bronchus intubation, tube displacement, inadequate ventilation and barotrauma.

22. a. **Elmslie–Trillat procedure.**
Surgical procedures for chronic patellofemoral instability are often used in combination and include soft tissue or bony procedures performed proximally, at the level of the joint or distal to it. A TT-TG distance of greater than 15 mm on CT suggests an increased Q-angle necessitating medial tibial tubercle transfer (Elmslie–Trillat). Unlike the Hauser technique, the Elmslie–Trillat does not involve posterior displacement which increases patellofemoral contact pressures contributing to pain and degeneration. Patellar alta is an indication for distal TT transfer. Trochlear dyplasia is recognized on lateral radiographs by the presence of the 'crossing sign' and may require a trochleoplasty to deepen and lateralize the trochlear groove. Lateral release is only indicated for isolated lateral patellar tilt and should be combined with another procedure if other factors are present. In the presence of a normal Q-angle, proximal soft tissue realignment procedures should be considered such as MPFL reconstruction and vastus medialis oblique (VMO) advancement.

23. c. **Homeobox genes**.
Limb buds are formed from mesoderm covered with surface ectoderm. The upper limb bud appears at 4 weeks post-fertilization and the lower limb bud appears two days later.
Two areas form within the mesoderm – the lateral mesoderm which forms bone, cartilage and connective tissues and the somite which forms the muscular elements. Homeobox (Hox) genes via fibroblast growth factors (FGFs) influence development of the apical ectodermal ridge (AER), which is responsible for proximal to distal growth. Hox gene abnormalities therefore lead to proximal/distal losses. The AER is a transient region of activity from which the digits develop. Separation of the digits occurs at around 50 days. Apoptosis under the influence of BMPs allows digits to separate and prevents webbing whereas noggins block apoptosis thereby preserving the webbing of the digits. The Sonic hedgehog genes control the zone of proliferating activity (ZPA) in the mesoderm that is responsible for radial to ulnar growth and differentiation, i.e. the little (fifth) finger from the thumb.

24. b. **There is an accepted and effective treatment**.
Neonatal hip instability is common; if instability persists, particularly when associated with anatomical dysplasia, true DDH develops. Clinical examination is less than 100% sensitive/specific and a missed diagnosis of DDH can lead to multiple invasive procedures and lifelong disability. Ultrasound screening in the neonatal period may therefore improve the accuracy of diagnosis leading to the provision of early treatment which is less invasive and of shorter duration with a greater likelihood of normal hip development. Although hip instability is commonly detectable in the newborn, most will resolve spontaneously without the need for treatment. However, there is no evidence proving the accuracy of ultrasound as a screening tool. Although ultrasound tends to lead to less invasive treatment of shorter duration, screening may lead to overtreatment. Not only is the evidence of the effectiveness of early non-invasive treatment lacking but non-invasive treatments such as the Pavlik harness are not without morbidity and carry a risk of AVN. Therefore, although ultrasound examination is a useful tool for assessing the infant hip prior to ossification, its use for screening remains controversial. It does not meet some of the criteria for a good screening test in that information on the natural history of the disease and the optimal treatment of DDH is lacking.
    Some countries provide generalized screening although this is not the case in the UK where selective screening of at-risk infants is performed.

25. d. **Presentation at 12–16 years**.
Tarsal coalition is due to failure of segmentation of the tarsal bones of the hind- and midfoot and can be partial or complete, fibrous, cartilaginous or bony. It is an autosomal dominant condition with a 20% incidence of multiple coalitions. Although congenital, symptoms occur when the coalition ossifies explaining why each type of coalition presents during a particular age range. Calcaneonavicular coalitions tend to present earlier between 8 and 12 years whereas talocalcaneal coalitions present later, at 12–16 years. Ossification causes loss of subtalar motion, adaptive shortening of the peronei and flatfeet; hence the term 'spastic peroneal flatfoot'. The typical presentation comprises recurrent ankle sprains, calf pain and flatfeet. The radiographic 'anteater sign' represents the elongated anterior process of the calcaneum in calcaneonavicular coalition whereas talar beaking can be seen whenever there is stiffness of the subtalar joint complex. Middle facet talocalcaneal coalition

produces the greatest subtalar stiffness, with a valgus hindfoot. Over time, the adaptive shortening of the peroneal tendons contributes to posterior facet arthrosis in the subtalar joint regardless of the type of coalition.

26. c. **Clinodactyly.**
The causes of congenital hand anomalies may be classified according to Swanson and the IFSSH (International Federation for Societies for Surgery of the Hand) system: failure of formation, failure of differentiation, duplication, hyperplasia, hypoplasia, amniotic bands, generalized dysplasias or combinations thereof.

Clinodactyly (failure of differentiation) is a fixed ulna bowing usually of the little finger.

Brachysyndactyly (failure of differentiation) means short digits with webbing between.

Camptodactyly (failure of differentiation) is characterized by fixed flexion deformity usually of the interphalangeal joints of the little fingers.

Acrosyndactyly is a form of constriction band syndrome which joins digits previously separated.

Symphalangism (failure of differentiation) is a congenital ankylosis usually affecting the proximal interphalangeal joints.

27. e. **Ischial tuberosity.**
The pelvic apophyses appear in early adolescence and fuse around age 14–16. Avulsions therefore occur most commonly in teenagers during sporting activities. Football and gymnastics are commonly associated with these injuries. Avulsion of the ischial tuberosity is the commonest type caused by sudden hip flexion with knee extension such as striking a football. The diagnosis is usually apparent on plain radiographs. Avulsion injuries are best treated conservatively with a gradual return to sporting activity after 3 months. Unrecognized avulsions may heal with abundant callus and can be misdiagnosed as bone tumours. The situation can be clarified with CT or MR imaging.

28. e. **Sharp's**
All of these lines on the anteroposterior (AP) pelvic radiograph are used to assess the degree of hip dysplasia/incongruence.

Hilgenreiner's line is made horizontally through the superior triradiate cartilage and serves as a reference for Perkin's line and for measuring the acetabular index.

Perkin's line is perpendicular to Hilgenreiner's at the superior edge of the ossified acetabulum. Normally, the femoral head should sit in the inferomedial quadrant at the intersection of these lines.

Shenton's line traces the lower edge of the pubis and the inferior aspect of the femoral neck. Any disruption to this line implies joint subluxation.

Wiberg's angle, known as the centre edge angle, is formed by the intersection of a line passing vertically upwards from the centre of the femoral head and a second line again passing from the centre of the head to the superior edge of the ossified acetabulum. This calculation is most reliable after age 5 due to increased ossification. A normal Wiberg's angle is $>25°$.

Sharps's line is an alternative method of measuring the acetabular angle. The more common method is to use Caffey's line drawn from the superior ossified acetabulum which forms an angle with Hilgenreiner's line at the superior margin of the triradiate cartilage. This method measures the superior acetabular angle that should be $<30°$ under age 2 and $<20°$ after age 2. Sharp's angle measures the inclination of the entire acetabulum. Sharp's angle is formed by the intersection of a horizontal line at the inferior teardrop and a line passing through it that joins the superolateral and inferomedial aspects of the bony socket. It is used after 9 months when the teardrop becomes visible radiologically. Normal infants should have a value of $<50°$ reducing to $<38°$ in adolescence.

29. a. Anterior shoulder dislocation.

Erb's palsy is the most common obstetric brachial plexus injury and the one with the best prognosis. It is caused by a traction injury at Erb's point: the union of the C5 and C6 nerve roots. The most commonly affected nerves are the axillary (supplying deltoid and teres minor), the suprascapular nerve (supplying the supraspinatus and infraspinatus muscles) and the musculocutaneous nerve (supplying biceps and brachialis muscles). Erb's palsy gives rise to the characteristic 'waiter's tip' deformity of shoulder adduction and internal rotation, elbow extension, forearm pronation and wrist flexion. Like other neuromuscular conditions in children, soft tissue contractures lead to secondary bony deformity and joint incongruence. In Erb's palsy, internal rotation of the shoulder caused by relative overactivity of subscapularis leads to dysplasia of the posterior glenoid and posterior (rather than anterior) instability.

30. a. Epiphyseal hyperplasia

Rubin classifies skeletal dysplasias according to their location of origin within the bone and whether due to over- or underactivity. Trevor's disease is also known as 'dysplasia epiphysealis hemimelica' and is due to hyperplasia within the epiphysis (epiphyseal osteochondroma). It is now more common for dysplasias to be diagnosed genetically rather than radiologically.

	Hypoplasia	Hyperplasia
Epiphysis	Spondyloepiphyseal dysplasia/multiple epiphyseal dysplasia	Trevor's disease
Physis	Achondroplasia	Enchondromatosis
Metaphysis	Osteopetrosis	Multiple hereditary exostoses
Diaphysis	Osteogenesis	Diaphyseal dysplasia

EMQs

1. 1. **c. PEX**. 2. **g. Core binding factor alpha-1 (CBFA1)**. 3. **b. X-linked recessive**.
Hypophosphataemic rickets is an example of an X-linked dominant condition where the defective PEX gene produces a non-functioning zinc-metalloproteinase. This enzyme usually breaks down FGF23 and its accumulation increases urinary excretion of phosphate and reduces alpha-1 hydroxylase activity. This accounts for the low serum phosphate and defective mineralization of bone. Males are often more affected than females due to the random inactivation of one of the X chromosomes in females.

The condition characterized by absent clavicles is cleidocranial dysostosis. The CBFA1 gene encodes a transcription factor for osteocalcin that regulates intramembranous ossification. The mutant state produces a proportionate dwarfism where the defining feature is partial or complete unilateral or bilateral aplasia of the clavicles and problems with formation of the skull bones.

Duchenne's muscular dystrophy is an X-linked recessive condition that presents with muscle weakness, difficulty walking and a Gower's sign on examination with pseudohypertrophy of some muscle groups. Gower's sign involves using the arms to splint the legs when rising from the floor due to weakness in the gluteal and quadriceps muscles. The gene defect results in virtually no production of the dystrophin protein that is responsible for maintaining muscle cell structure; its absence leads to cell death. In Becker's muscular dystrophy, a similar genetic defect exists that results in the production of defective dystrophin.

2. 1. **h. Ratliff**. 2. **f. Harcke**. 3. **a. Achtermann and Kalamchi**.
Avascular necrosis (AVN) may occur following hip trauma in children due to the reliance on end arteries. Ratliff classifies AVN of the proximal femur according to the degree of involvement. Type I signifies involvement of the entire head and carries the worst prognosis, type II signifies partial head involvement and type III signifies involvement of the neck. Kalamchi and MacEwen is a classification of AVN following DDH.

Both Harcke and Graf systems can be used to assess developmental dysplasia of the hip (DDH) using ultrasound. The Harcke system is a dynamic test of stability and employs transverse plane imaging. Graf is a static test using coronal plane imaging to determine morphology and coverage. The most important aspect of neonatal DDH is the associated joint instability so dynamic testing is often considered to be an integral part of the assessment process. Crowe is a radiographic classification of the degree of subluxation/ dislocation in DDH.

Fibular hemimelia is the most obvious post-axial limb deficiency and used the Achtermann and Kalamchi classification:

Type I is a hypoplastic fibula where the proximal physis lies below the proximal tibial physis and the distal physis is above the talar dome.

Type II involves loss of 30–50% of the fibula where the distal end does not contribute to ankle stability.

Type III involves complete fibula loss.

Aiken classifies proximal femoral focal deficiency (PFFD) which may be a component part of fibular hemimelia.

3. 1. **f. Sacral agenesis**. 2. **e. Sprengel's shoulder**. 3. **h. Clinodactyly**.
Although maternal diabetes may be associated with other congenital anomalies, there is a very strong correlation with sacral agenesis.

The omovertebral bone is a cartilaginous or osseous bridge between the superomedial scapula and the lower cervical spine, seen in Sprengel's shoulder.

An ulnar bowing of the little finger identified on antenatal ultrasound, indicating clinodactyly, is associated with a significantly increased risk of a chromosomal anomaly particularly Trisomy 21 (in 80%).

4. 1. **i. Salter–Harris VI**. 2. **j. Salter–Harris V**. 3. **g. Salter–Harris IV**.
Salter and Harris originally described five types of injury to the physis although nine types are now recognized following additions by others to the classification. A type VI injury, added by Mercer Rang (1969) involves damage to the perichondral ring which frequently leads to a bony bridge formation and angular deformity.

Acetabular fractures in children can involve the triradiate cartilage causing subsequent acetabular dysplasia. Bucholz *et al* suggest that such injuries are equivalent either to a Salter–Harris I, II or V with the latter having the poorest outcome due to growth arrest.

The Lauge-Hansen classification of adult ankle fractures has been modified by Dias and Tachdjian in children. A supination-inversion injury shears off the medial malleolus vertically through the physis involving both epiphysis and metaphysis, i.e. a Salter–Harris IV injury.

5. 1. **i. Osteopetrosis**. 2. **d. Hypothyroidism**. 3. **e. Vitamin D-resistant rickets**.
In osteopetrosis, due to decreased osteoclastic resorption, dense bone accumulates in the marrow space inhibiting haematopoiesis giving rise to anaemia. Bone marrow transplant may be required in certain cases.

True bilateral Perthes disease has an incidence of approximately 10%. The differential diagnosis includes epiphyseal dysplasias (spondyloepiphyseal dysplasia (SED), multiple epiphyseal dysplasia (MED)) and hypothyroidism. Hypothyroidism leads to growth retardation and delayed appearance of ossification centres that may fragment. It is also associated with a higher incidence of slipped upper femoral epiphysis (SUFE) and avascular necrosis (AVN).

Vitamin D-resistant rickets, also known as familial hypophosphataemic rickets, is an X-linked dominant condition, characterized by large renal losses of phosphate and reduced response to vitamin D. It is the commonest bone mineralization defect.

6. 1. **b. Ewing's sarcoma**. 2. **f. Fibrous dysplasia**. 3. **a. Osteoid osteoma**.
Like other primitive neuroectodermal tumours, Ewing's sarcoma demonstrates the translocation t (11:22). It is a highly malignant tumour, occurring in the first two decades of life.

Fibrous dysplasia is characterized by growth of fibro-osseous tissue that cannot mature into lamellar bone. It may therefore present with pathological fractures. Most commonly monostotic affecting the proximal femur but can be polyostotic with variable distribution. McCune–Albright's syndrome refers to fibrous dysplasia associated with precocious puberty and café-au-lait spots. Mazabraud's syndrome refers to fibrous dysplasia associated with intramuscular myxoma.

Osteoid osteoma is a benign condition usually affecting the cortex of the diaphysis or metaphysis of the femur or found in the spine. A small nidus is seen often surrounded by a dense sclerotic reactive zone on plain films (less than 2 cm in diameter).

7. 1. **j. Myaesthenia gravis.** 2. **c. Charcot–Marie–Tooth disease.** 3. **d. Friedreich's ataxia.** Myaesthenia gravis is an auto-immune disease where circulating antibodies bind to and inactivate acetylcholine receptors at the post-synaptic side of the neuromuscular junction. Because Botox (botulinum toxin) inhibits release of acetylcholine from the presynaptic side, its use is contraindicated in myasthenia gravis.

PMP22 stands for peripheral myelin protein 22 and it is defective in Charcot–Marie–Tooth disease. It is an integral membrane protein expressed by Schwann cells and an important component of the myelin sheath. Affected individuals suffer both sensory and motor losses.

Friedreich's ataxia is caused by mitochondrial dysfunction. A silent frataxin protein allows an accumulation of iron in the cytoplasm around mitochondria thereby defunctioning them. Nerve and muscle cells are particularly sensitive to this and the effect on cerebellar neurons gives rise to the characteristic ataxic signs.

8. 1. **d. Group B streptococci.** 2. **e. *Staphylococcus aureus*.** 3. **e. *Staphylococcus aureus*.** Group B streptococci is a common commensal in the maternal vagina and rectum and can be passed on to the baby during delivery. It is responsible for osteoarticular infection in the neonatal age group. The risk of group B streptococci infection increases if there is delay in delivery after artificial rupture of the membranes.

Staphylococcus aureus is the commonest pathogen in a child of 5. The HiB vaccine has made infection with *Haemophilus influenzae* much less common.

Although patients with sickle cell disease have a greater chance of succumbing to atypical pathogens such as salmonella, infections with *Staphylococcus aureus* are more common.

9. 1. **j. Pes cavovarus.** 2. **a. Congenital vertical talus.** 3. **b. Skewfoot.** Pes cavovarus is characterized by a varus hindfoot and a high arch with a plantarflexed first ray. The Coleman block test determines flexibility of the hindfoot by placing a block under its lateral border. If a stiff hindfoot exists, then a valgus calcaneal osteotomy is required.

Congenital vertical talus gives the appearance of an equinovalgus foot. An oblique talus differs in that the talonavicular dislocation reduces with plantarflexion and the hindfoot is not usually in equinus.

In a skewfoot, the valgus hindfoot is associated with an adducted forefoot, which becomes worse if the hindfoot is corrected without acknowledging this relationship. The pes planovalgus (the common flatfoot) has an abducted forefoot that is pronated.

10. 1. **e. Spondylolysis** 2. **h. Flat back syndrome.** 3. **a. Scheuermann's disease** Spondylolysis, also known as a pars interarticularis fracture, occurs classically in gymnasts due to repeated hyperextension of the spine. The oblique radiograph of the lumbar spine shows the fracture through the 'Scottie dog's neck' (Lachapelle).

Flat back syndrome is an iatrogenic flattening of the lumbar lordosis following surgical correction of a scoliosis without considering the multiplanar nature of the deformity.

It occurs when distraction osteosynthesis is placed without regard to the sagittal deformity: reducing a lumbar lordosis with a thoracic kyphosis proximally produces difficulty in standing up straight.

Scheuermann's disease is a thoracic kyphosis, which is often self-limiting and characterized by anterior wedging of the vertebral bodies, and is a form of juvenile osteochondritis.

11. 1.   **j. Bone within a bone.** 2. **i. Sagging rope.** 3. **a. Fallen fragment.**
Bone within a bone is seen with osteopetrosis, which results from decreased osteoclastic activity secondary to carbonic anhydrase deficiency. The relative overactivity of osteoblasts results in thick, dense but brittle bone. The bone within a bone appearance results from the cyclical activity of the cells where alternating layers of dense bone and normal bone are laid down.

The sagging rope sign is seen with growth disturbance of the proximal femur secondary to AVN, which leads to overgrowth and flattening of the femoral head. Radiographically, the overhanging femoral head projects a line onto the metaphysis which give the appearance of a sagging rope. Gage's sign is associated with AVN due to Perthes disease and is often defined as a V-shaped defect in the lateral metaphysis and is a 'head-at-risk' sign (but this is not what Gage described!)

The fallen fragment sign is seen with a unicameral or simple bone cyst. This is usually asymptomatic until a pathological fracture occurs. The fallen fragment represents a piece of cortex that has fallen into the dependent part of the fluid-filled cyst. This sign is also called the 'fallen leaf' sign.

12. 1.   **f. Snapping fascia lata.** 2. **d. Femoroacetabular impingement.** 3. **c. Slipped upper femoral epiphysis (SUFE).**
The Ober test demonstrates tightness in fascia lata. The patient lies on their non-affected side, the hip is abducted, extended, externally rotated and then allowed to adduct. The fascia lata is tight if there is resistance to passive adduction in this position, and this is likely to be the case in snapping fascia lata.

Femoroacetabular impingement may occur secondary to several different childhood hip conditions; it leads to superior acetabular damage at the chondrolabral junction.

Trethowan's sign is positive when Klein's line (drawn along the superior femoral neck on a plain anteroposterior (AP) pelvic radiograph) does not intersect with any part of the lateral epiphysis; this is seen with SUFE.

13. 1.   **b. Pemberton.** 2. **h. Chiari.** 3. **a. Ganz.**
The Pemberton is an incomplete transiliac osteotomy equivalent to Dega's osteotomy that hinges on the triradiate cartilage. The osteotomy begins 10–15 mm above the anterior interior iliac spine (AIIS) and curves posteriorly ending at the ilioischial limb of the triradiate cartilage. It is inherently stable as the posterior column remains intact. The acetabular volume is reduced in this procedure.

Both the Chiari and shelf procedures are salvage techniques to gain lateral cover. The shelf involves applying cortical bone graft to the anterolateral ilium whereas the Chiari osteotomy is a complete iliac osteotomy where the acetabular fragment is displaced medially.

The Ganz, also known as the periacetabular or Bernese osteotomy, is made close to the acetabulum allowing significant correction of acetabular alignment in patients who are skeletally mature. The osteotomy is inherently more stable than some as the posterior column is intact.

14. 1. **g. 7**. 2. **h. 8**. 3. **j. 10**.

The ossification centres of the elbow appear at years 1, 3, 5, 7, 9 and 11. Using the mnemonic 'CRITOL' (or CRITOE) to determine their sequence of appearance, a child with a visible trochlear ossification centre is around age 7.

Erb's palsy affects C5 and 6 whereas Klumpke's affects C8 and T1. This affects the wrist flexors and the intrinsic muscles. The presence of a Horner's syndrome (T1) is a poor prognostic sign.

By definition, an intralesional resection has a local recurrence rate of 100%, a marginal excision 25% and wide excision a risk of approximately 10%.

15. 1. **b. Inferior patellar**. 2. **h. Iliac crest**. 3. **a. Medial epicondyle**.

Sinding-Larsen–Johansson is similar to Osgood–Schlatter's disease but represents a traction tendinitis of the proximal patellar tendon (inferior patella) with de novo calcification rather than a traction apophysitis.

The iliac crest apophysis can become avulsed during tennis serves due to sudden contraction of the abdominal wall muscles opposed by the gluteal or tensor fascia lata muscles.

The medial epicondyle apophysis appears at age 5 years, although it is commonly avulsed between 9 and 14 years following a valgus-producing force at the elbow. It is commonly associated with elbow dislocation and can become incarcerated within the joint requiring extraction and fixation.

Selected references

Aguilar JA, Paley D, Paley J et al. Clinical validation of the multiplier method for predicting limb length discrepancy and outcome of epiphysiodesis, part II. *J Pediatr Orthop* 2005; **25**(2): 192–6.

Bucholz RW, Ezaki M, Ogden JA. Injury to the acetabular triradiate physeal cartilage. *J Bone Joint Surg Am* 1982; **64**(4): 600–9.

Clohisy JC, Carlisle JC, Beaulé PE et al. A systematic approach to the plain radiographic evaluation of the young adult hip. *J Bone Joint Surg Am* 2008; **90** (Suppl 4): 47–66.

Herring-JA, Kim-HT, Browne-R. Legg Calvé Perthes disease. Part I: Classification of radiographs with use of the modified lateral pillar and Stulberg classifications. *J Bone Joint Surg Am* 2004; **86**(10): 2103–20.

Kocher MS, Mandiga R, Zurakowski D, Barnewolt C, Kasser JR. Validation of a clinical prediction rule for the differentiation between septic arthritis and transient synovitis of the hip in children. *J Bone Joint Surg Am* 2004; **86**: 1629–35.

Kocher MS, Zurakowski D, Kasser JR. Differentiating between septic arthritis and transient synovitis of the hip in children: an evidence-based clinical prediction algorithm. *J Bone Joint Surg Am* 1999; **81**(12): 1662–70.

Menelaus MB. Correction of leg length discrepancy by epiphyseal arrest. *J Bone Joint Surg Br* 1966; **48**(2): 336–9.

Moon ES, Mehlman CT. Risk factors for avascular necrosis after femoral neck fractures in children. 25 Cincinnati cases and meta-analysis of 360 cases. *J Orthop Trauma* 2006; **20**: 323–9.

Mulford JS, Wakeley CJ, Eldridge JDJ. Assessment and management of chronic patellofemoral instability. *J Bone Joint Surg Br* 2007; **89**(6): 709–16.

Woolacott NF, Puhan MA, Steurer J, Kleijnen J. Ultrasonography in screening for developmental dysplasia of the hip in newborns: systematic review. *BMJ* 2005; **330**: 1413.

MCQs

1. **Concerning Pipkin's classification of femoral head and neck fractures, which of the following is not true?**
   a. Posterior dislocation of the hip with fracture of the femoral head caudal to the fovea centralis is a type I fracture.
   b. A type III fracture is rare, in conjunction with femoral neck fracture.
   c. Posterior dislocation of the hip with fracture of the femoral head cephalad to the fovea centralis is a type II fracture.
   d. A femoral head fracture with associated fracture of the acetabulum is a type III fracture.
   e. A and D.

2. **Considering Schatzker's classification of fractures of the tibial plateau, which of the following statements is false?**
   a. Type I fractures are wedge fractures of the lateral plateau, displaced or undisplaced.
   b. Type III fractures show depression of the lateral plateau without an associated wedge fracture.
   c. Type II fractures are often seen in patients whose average age is over 50.
   d. Anterior cruciate ligament injuries are commonly seen in type V and VI injuries.
   e. A type V fracture consists of a wedge fracture of the medial and lateral plateaux with metaphyseal–diaphyseal discontinuity.

3. **Which of the following statements is incorrect regarding ankle fractures?**
   a. On a mortise view, the tibiofibular overlap should normally be more than 4 mm.
   b. A Maisonneuve fracture is a high fibular fracture and involves disruption of syndesmosis.
   c. A Dupuytren's fracture is a fracture-dislocation with a high fibular fracture.
   d. On an anteroposterior (AP) radiograph, the medial clear space should be less than 4 mm.
   e. The talocrural angle can be used to assess shortening.

Postgraduate Orthopaedics, ed. Kesavan Sri-Ram. Published by Cambridge University Press.
© Cambridge University Press 2012.

4. **A previously healthy 41-year-old man suffers a minimally displaced distal radius fracture and is treated in a cast for 4 weeks. He presents 14 weeks later with dorsal wrist pain. What is the most likely diagnosis?**
   a. Rupture of the extensor pollicis longus (EPL) tendon.
   b. Rupture of the extensor indicis proprius (EIP) tendon.
   c. Missed scaphoid fracture.
   d. De Quervain's tenosynovitis.
   e. Arthritis of the first carpometacarpal joint.

5. **Which of the following inflammatory mediators has been most closely associated with the magnitude of the inflammatory response to blunt trauma and with the development of multiple organ dysfunction syndrome (MODS)?**
   a. Interleukin-1 (IL-1).
   b. Beta human chorionic gonadotrophin (ß-HCG).
   c. Tumour necrosis factor beta (TGF-ß).
   d. Tumour necrosis factor alpha (TNF-α).
   e. Interleukin-6 (IL-6).

6. **Which of the following is true regarding scapholunate dissociation?**
   a. A scapholunate distance of more than 1 mm is diagnostic.
   b. An MRI scan is mandatory.
   c. The Madonna sign is diagnostic.
   d. The cortical ring sign is produced by cortex of distal pole of palmar flexed scaphoid.
   e. On the lateral view, a scapholunate angle of >40–45° suggests scapholunate dissociation.

7. **With reference to injuries around the elbow, which of the following statements is false?**
   a. A type III coronoid fracture involves more than half of the coronoid.
   b. The anterior, oblique portion of the medial collateral ligament is the primary stabilizer of the elbow to valgus stress.
   c. The lateral collateral ligament is a stabilizer of the elbow to varus stress.
   d. The combination of dislocation, coronoid fracture and radial head fracture is known colloquially as 'the terrible triad'.
   e. The posterior, transverse portion of medial collateral ligament is the primary stabilizer of the elbow to valgus stress.

8. **'Functional bracing' for a humeral diaphyseal fracture relies upon which type of bone healing?**
   a. Enchondral ossification.
   b. Primary bone healing.
   c. Haversian remodelling.
   d. Healing with osteons.
   e. Appositional bone growth.

9. **An 86-year-old man falls and sustains a minimally displaced proximal humerus fracture. What is the best way to manage him?**
   a. Physiotherapy and passive range of motion, 10 days following the injury.
   b. Immobilization for 4 weeks in a sling.

   c. Physiotherapy the following day, with range of motion exercises.
   d. Intramedullary nail fixation.
   e. Urgent open reduction and locking plate fixation.

10. **When considering spinal fractures, which of the following is true?**
   a. AO type A fractures are rotational injuries.
   b. AO type B fractures are rotational injuries.
   c. Finger abduction is under the control of the C7 nerve root.
   d. A Chance fracture is a two-column extension injury.
   e. In a thoracic cord injury, the return of the bulbocavernosus reflex signals the termination of spinal shock.

11. **A 30-year-old woman is involved in a road traffic accident and is found to have a pelvic symphysis separation of 4 cm and a sacral fracture. She undergoes a normal secondary survey and is haemodynamically stable. Definitive fixation should involve which of the following?**
   a. Skeletal traction for 3 months.
   b. Internal fixation of the symphysis pubis with anterior external fixation.
   c. Internal fixation of the symphysis pubis and internal fixation of the sacrum.
   d. Posterior only external fixation.
   e. Anterior only external fixation.

12. **When predicting the outcome after distal radius fractures, which of the following is false?**
   a. Age is an important factor if predicting early instability of minimally displaced fractures.
   b. Age is an important factor if predicting late instability of minimally displaced fractures.
   c. In the prediction of malunion, the presence or absence of comminution is not an important factor.
   d. Age is an important factor if predicting malunion.
   e. The dorsal angle at presentation is not important in predicting malunion in displaced fractures.

13. **When considering traumatic scapulothoracic dissociation, which of the following is false?**
   a. The brachial plexus injury is most predictive of outcome.
   b. It is nearly always a high-energy injury.
   c. 80% will also have a clavicle fracture.
   d. 10% occur in motorcyclists.
   e. It results from a massive traction force to the upper limb.

14. **An 11-year-old girl sustains a closed femoral shaft fracture, which is then treated with an anterograde intramedullary nail via a piriformis fossa entry point. In follow-up, she is noted to have collapse of the femoral head. This is most likely due to?**
   a. Missed concurrent subcapital fracture.
   b. Infection.
   c. Pressure changes within the capsule of the hip joint.

    d. Perthes disease.
    e. Injury to the lateral ascending vessels of the femoral neck.

15. **Concerning intramembranous ossification, which of the following is true?**
    a. It occurs in all long bone fractures.
    b. It is affected in Hurler's syndrome.
    c. It is responsible for bone formation in distraction osteogenesis.
    d. It is associated with osteons.
    e. It is a feature of callus in physeal fractures.

16. **In relation to fractures of the intercondylar eminence of the tibia, which of the following statements is true?**
    a. The flexion deformity usually seen is caused by the impingement of the displaced fragment.
    b. The injury is more likely visualized on the anteroposterior (AP) radiograph.
    c. The highest incidence is seen between the ages 8 and 13.
    d. Aspiration of a tense haemarthrosis is not advised.
    e. In a type II fracture, bony union is not possible without reduction manoeuvres.

17. **What effect would doubling the diameter of a solid intramedullary nail have on its torsional rigidity?**
    a. No effect.
    b. Increase by 2-fold.
    c. Increase by 4-fold.
    d. Increase by 8-fold.
    e. Increase by 16-fold.

18. **Which indication would be considered the best reason for the use of a locking plate in the treatment of a diaphyseal radial fracture?**
    a. A need for early return to function.
    b. A stable fracture configuration.
    c. A paediatric patient.
    d. An open fracture.
    e. Marked osteopaenia.

19. **Which of the following patients would you expect to fare better with operative management of a displaced calcaneal fracture?**
    a. Young woman, heavy smoker.
    b. 60-year-old woman, otherwise healthy.
    c. Young woman, injured hill-running.
    d. Healthy man, injured at work.
    e. Young healthy woman with bilateral fractures.

20. **A 31-year-old woman has fracture-dislocation at C5–C6. A clavicle fracture is noted on an otherwise normal chest X-ray. Her pulse is 45, blood pressure is 83/40 mmHg and respiratory rate is 28. An abdominal ultrasound is negative. What type of shock is most likely in this patient?**
    a. Haemorrhagic.
    b. Septic.

c. Neurogenic.

d. Spinal.

e. Tension pneumothorax.

21. **Which complication below is most likely following open reduction and fixation of a Lisfranc injury?**

    a. Non-union.

    b. Failure of metalwork.

    c. Infection.

    d. Arthritis.

    e. Avascular necrosis.

22. **With reference to the management of open fractures, which of the following is true?**

    a. All wounds should undergo immediate surgical exploration.

    b. For haemorrhage control, a tourniquet should never be used.

    c. In compartment syndrome a difference of 30 mmHg or less between the measured pressure and the systolic blood pressure is a reasonable threshold for decompression.

    d. It is the 10 cm perforator from the posterior tibial artery, medially which is usually the largest and most reliable for distally based fascio-cutaneous flaps.

    e. Absent or reduced plantar sensation at initial presentation is an indication for primary amputation.

23. **Which of the following is true of sternoclavicular dislocations?**

    a. Posterior sternoclavicular dislocations are more common than anterior.

    b. The anterior capsular ligament is the most important structure for anterior-posterior stability.

    c. On a serendipity view radiograph, an anterior dislocation would show the affected clavicle above the contralateral clavicle.

    d. All traumatic sternoclavicular dislocations need reduction.

    e. The posterior sternoclavicular ligament is the primary restraint to superior displacement of the medial clavicle.

24. **A 6-year-old has a posteriorly displaced supracondylar fracture, with absent pulses, but a warm, pink hand. What is the optimal management?**

    a. Immediate reduction of the fracture in the emergency department.

    b. Open reduction with immediate exploration by a vascular surgeon.

    c. Closed reduction in theatre, with reassessment of the vascularity.

    d. Urgent brachial angiography.

    e. Exploration by a vascular surgeon followed by external fixation.

25. **Which of the following is not true regarding the anterior ilioinguinal approach to the pelvis?**

    a. The first window is the internal iliac fossa bounded medially by the iliopsoas.

    b. The second window gives access to the pelvic brim and quadrilateral plate.

    c. The corona mortis may extend over the anterior column in the area of the superior pubic ramus.

    d. Inadequate closure of the floor of the inguinal canal may lead to an indirect inguinal hernia.

e. This approach will allow visualization of the interior of the iliac wing, anterior sacroiliac joint, entire anterior column and pubic symphysis.

26. **Which of the following is false with reference to the Kocher–Langenbeck approach for pelvic fractures?**
    a. It is recommended for isolated posterior column injuries.
    b. The superior neurovascular bundle is at greatest risk during exposure of the greater sciatic notch.
    c. The pudendal nerve is at risk as it enters the pelvis through the greater sciatic notch.
    d. Branches of the medial femoral circumflex artery are within the quadratus femoris muscle.
    e. It has been associated with abductor weakness.

27. **Which of the following would not increase the stability of an external fixator?**
    a. Increasing the diameter of the pins.
    b. Increasing the distance between the rods and the bone.
    c. Increasing the number of pins.
    d. Increasing the space between the pins.
    e. Placing pins in different planes.

28. **Which of the following is not a type of acetabular fracture according to the Judet and Letournel classification?**
    a. Posterior column.
    b. Anterior column and posterior hemitransverse.
    c. Posterior wall and posterior column.
    d. Posterior column and posterior hemitransverse.
    e. Posterior wall and transverse.

29. **Which of the following best describes a Jones fracture?**
    a. Avulsion flake fracture from the base of the fifth metatarsal.
    b. Proximal metaphyseal fracture of the fifth metatarsal at the level of the tarsometatarsal joint.
    c. Fracture at the metaphyseal–diaphyseal junction of the fifth metatarsal at the level of the fourth–fifth intermetatarsal articulation.
    d. Fracture at the proximal diaphysis of the fifth metatarsal distal to the level of the fourth–fifth intermetatarsal articulation.
    e. Fracture at the distal diaphysis of the fifth metatarsal distal to the level of the fourth–fifth intermetatarsal articulation.

30. **Which of the following is not a contraindication to functional brace treatment for a humeral shaft fracture?**
    a. Ipsilateral radial shaft fracture.
    b. Associated radial nerve palsy.
    c. Associated brachial plexus palsy.
    d. Uncooperative patient.
    e. Ipsilateral clavicle fracture.

EMQs

1. **The small fragment osteosynthesis set**
   a. 1.9 mm
   b. 2.0 mm
   c. 2.1 mm
   d. 2.3 mm
   e. 2.4 mm
   f. 2.5 mm
   g. 2.7 mm
   h. 2.8 mm
   i. 3.0 mm
   j. 3.4 mm
   k. 3.5 mm
   l. 4.0 mm

Which of the options above is best described in each of the following statements? Each option may be used once, more than once or not at all.
   1. This is the drill bit size used for a 3.5 mm cortical screw.
   2. This is the tap size used for a 3.5 mm cortical screw.
   3. This is the drill bit size used for a 3.5 mm locking screw.

2. **Scoring and grading in relation to trauma**
   a. B1
   b. C2
   c. B3
   d. 2
   e. 4
   f. 8
   g. 9
   h. B2
   i. 10
   j. 11
   k. 12
   l. C3

Which of the options above is best described in each of the following statements? Each option may be used once, more than once or not at all.
   1. The Mirel's score in a patient with an intertrochanteric fracture who had moderate pain through an area of lysis from a metastasis, which occupied less than one-third of the width of the bone.
   2. The Vancouver classification for a fracture around the stem of a loose hip prosthesis with severe bone loss.
   3. The Oestern and Tscherne classification of a closed radial shaft fracture with an overlying superficial abrasion.

3. **Cervical spine injuries**
   a. Type I odontoid fracture
   b. Pseudosubluxation

  c. Bilateral facet dislocation
  d. C1–C2 rotatory subluxation
  e. Hangman's fracture
  f. Unilateral facet dislocation
  g. Type II odontoid fracture
  h. Jefferson's fracture
  i. Type III odontoid fracture

Which of the options above is best described in each of the following statements? Each option may be used once, more than once or not at all.
1. A 19-year-old presents with a very painful neck following an axial compression injury.
2. A 7-year-old boy falls down some stairs. He has mild neck pain. His lateral cervical spine X-ray shows 4 mm translation of C2 on C3.
3. An 18-year-old falls down some stairs. He has mild neck pain. His lateral cervical spine X-ray shows a 'bow tie' sign.

4. **Upper limb trauma**
  a. Galleazzi fracture
  b. Monteggia fracture
  c. Barton's fracture
  d. Rolando fracture
  e. Bennett's fracture
  d. Smith's fracture
  f. Colles fracture
  g. Essex-Lopresti injury
  h. Stener lesion

Which of the options above is best described in each of the following statements? Each option may be used once, more than once or not at all.
1. This is an injury that is classified by Bado.
2. This is a Y- or T-shaped intra-articular fracture described in 1910.
3. This involves dislocation of the distal radioulnar joint and fracture of the radial head.

5. **Pelvic and hip radiographs**
  a. Shenton's line
  b. Nelaton's line
  c. Klein's line
  d. Hilgenreiner's line
  e. Trethowan's line
  f. Perkin's line
  g. Ilioischial line
  h. Iliopectineal line
  i. Northern line
  j. Iliopubic line

Which of the options above is best described in each of the following statements? Each option may be used once, more than once or not at all.

1. This demarcates the medial border of the posterior column of the acetabulum.
2. This is a curvilinear line along the inferior margin of the superior pubic ramus which continues along the inferior border of the femoral neck.
3. This is a line drawn between the two tri-radiate cartilages.

6. **Considering spinal cord injuries**
   a. Brown-Séquard syndrome
   b. Central cord syndrome
   c. Complete transection of the cord
   d. Conus medullaris syndrome
   e. Anterior cord syndrome
   f. Tabes dorsalis
   g. Tethered cord syndrome
   h. Posterior cord syndrome
   i. None of the above

Which of the options above is best described in each of the following statements? Each option may be used once, more than once or not at all.

1. Only 10–15% of patients demonstrate functional recovery following this.
2. This injury is associated with the best prognosis.
3. This produces contralateral muscle paralysis and ipsilateral hyperaesthesia to pain and temperature.

7. **Injuries to peripheral nerves**
   a. Superficial radial nerve
   b. Posterior interosseous nerve
   c. Median nerve
   d. Anterior interosseous nerve
   e. Ulnar nerve
   f. Axillary nerve
   g. Medial cutaneous nerve of the forearm
   h. Medial cutaneous nerve of the arm
   i. Musculocutaneous nerve
   j. Thoracodorsal nerve
   k. Suprascapular nerve
   l. Lateral pectoral nerve
   m. Medial pectoral nerve

Which of the options above is best described in each of the following statements? Each option may be used once, more than once or not at all.

1. A 23-year-old man is stabbed in the volar aspect of the forearm. He is unable to flex his index finger distal interphalangeal joint, but can flex the ring finger one.
2. A 23-year-old man is stabbed in the volar aspect of the forearm. He has poor function in his hand, and is offered a Camitz transfer after he fails to recover.

3. A 31-year-old has a radial head fracture fixed, under an interscalene block. Post-operatively he has persistent numbness over the lateral aspect of the forearm.

8. **Mangled Extremity Severity Score (MESS)**
   a. 2
   b. 3
   c. 4
   d. 5
   e. 7
   f. 9
   g. 10
   h. 11
   i. 12
   j. 13
   k. 14

Which of the options above is best described in each of the following statements? Each option may be used once, more than once or not at all.
   1. A 74-year-old man who has slipped on a wet floor half an hour ago presents with a blood pressure of 100/60 mmHg and pulse of 64. He has a closed tibia fracture in a normally perfused leg, but with reduced pulses.
   2. A 74-year-old man who has slipped on a wet floor 8 hours ago presents with a blood pressure of 100/60 mmHg and pulse of 64. He has a hip fracture in a normally perfused leg, but with reduced pulses.
   3. A 44-year-old female is shot by a high velocity rifle resulting in a cold, insensate lower leg and an open tibial fracture. Her blood pressure is recorded an hour after the injury as 80/60 mmHg despite aggressive fluid resuscitation.

9. **Injuries to the elbow**
   a. Supracondylar fracture
   b. Lateral condyle fracture
   c. Medial condyle fracture
   d. Coronoid fracture
   e. Radial head fracture
   f. Radial neck fracture
   g. Olecranon fracture
   h. Capitellum fracture
   i. Radial head dislocation
   j. Elbow dislocation
   k. Intercondylar fracture
   l. D and E
   m. D and F
   n. E and H
   o. D and H
   p. E and F

Which of the options above is best described in each of the following statements? Each option may be used once, more than once or not at all.
1. A 22-year-old dislocates his left elbow. His radiographs suggest he has a 'terrible triad' injury of the elbow.
2. A 23-year-old falls over and injures his right elbow. Radiographs show a Kocher–Lorenz injury.
3. A 44-year-old falls over and presents with a painful elbow and absent distal pulses.

10. **Classifications of fractures**
    a. Mayfield
    b. Tile
    c. Garden
    d. Young–Burgess
    e. Damschen
    f. Essex-Lopresti
    g. Mason
    h. AO
    i. Bado
    j. Frykman
    k. Gustillo

Which of the options above is best described in each of the following statements? Each option may be used once, more than once or not at all.
1. A force-vector mechanistic classification of pelvic injuries.
2. A proposed classification for scapulothoracic dissociation.
3. A classification of radial head fractures.

11. **Techniques of fracture management**
    a. Reamed intramedullary nailing with dynamic interlocking
    b. Closed reduction and plaster immobilization
    c. Unreamed intramedullary nailing with dynamic interlocking
    d. Retrograde flexible intramedullary nailing
    e. Anterograde flexible intramedullary nailing
    f. Closed reduction and K-wire fixation
    g. Unreamed intramedullary nailing with static interlocking
    h. Reamed intramedullary nailing with static interlocking
    i. Compression plating
    j. Observation

Which of the options above is best described in each of the following statements? Each option may be used once, more than once or not at all.
1. A 34-year-old man suffers an isolated, closed diaphyseal femoral fracture and is haemodynamically stable.
2. A 9-year-old boy presents with a displaced diaphyseal femoral fracture.
3. A 7-year-old girl sustains a fracture of her proximal tibial metaphysis and is treated with a period of immobilization 9 months earlier. She presents in clinic with very anxious parents who are worried she is developing 'knock knees'.

12. Compartments

a. 1
b. 2
c. 3
d. 4
e. 5
f. 6
g. 7
h. 8
i. 9
j. 10
k. 11
l. 12

Which of the options above is best described in each of the following statements? Each option may be used once, more than once or not at all.

1. The number of compartments in the lower leg.
2. The number of compartments in the hand.
3. The number of compartments in the forearm.

13. Injuries around the knee

a. Pellegrini–Stieda
b. Hoffa
c. Segond
d. Myers–McKeever
e. Schatzker
f. Patella sleeve
g. Sindig-Larsen–Johanssen
h. Osgood–Schlatter
i. Bipartite patella

Which of the options above is best described in each of the following statements? Each option may be used once, more than once or not at all.

1. A 33-year-old presents with knee pain. Radiographs show mineralization of the proximal part of the medial collateral ligament.
2. A 24-year-old injures his knee. Radiographs show a condylar fracture in the coronal plane.
3. A 23-year-old injures his knee. Clinical examination reveals a positive pivot shift test.

14. Surgical approaches in trauma

a. Kocher's
b. Kocher–Langenbeck
c. Henry's
d. Thompson's
e. Triceps split
f. Deltopectoral

   g. Smith–Petersen
   h. Southern
   i.   Lateral parapatellar
   j. Medial parapatellar

Which of the options above is best described in each of the following statements? Each option may be used once, more than once or not at all.
1. Exploits an internervous plane between the femoral and superior gluteal nerves.
2. Exploits an internervous plane between the radial and median nerves.
3. Will involve encountering the ascending branch of the lateral femoral circumflex artery.

15. **Head injury**
   a. Concussion
   b. Cerebral haemorrhage
   c. Epidural haemorrhage
   d. Subdural haemorrhage
   e. Subarachnoid haemorrhage
   f. Cerebral contusion
   g. Diffuse axonal injury
   h. Depressed skull fracture
   i.   Basilar skull fracture

Which of the options above is best described in each of the following statements? Each option may be used once, more than once or not at all.
1. A 41-year-old man sustains a head injury. Clinical examination reveals Battle's sign.
2. A 31-year-old sustains a head injury and his scan reveals bleeding from the middle meningeal artery.
3. A 31-year-old sustains a head injury and his scan reveals bleeding from the bridging veins.

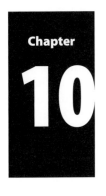

Chapter

10

Trauma: Answers

Paul Whittingham-Jones, Kesavan Sri-Ram and Dennis Edwards

MCQs

1. **d. A femoral head fracture with associated fracture of the acetabulum is a type III fracture.**

Femoral head fractures are rare, and are almost always associated with hip dislocations; approximately 7% of posterior hip dislocations are associated with a femoral head fracture. Posterior hip dislocations are classified according to Thompson/Epstein:

I– with or without a minor fracture

II– with a large single fracture of the posterior acetabular rim

III– with comminution of the rim of the acetabulum, with or without a major fragment

IV– with a fracture of the acetabular floor

V– with a fracture of the femoral head

The type V injuries are further classified by Pipkin, according to the femoral head fracture:

I– below fovea centralis

II– above fovea centralis

III– I or II with associated femoral neck fracture

IV– I, II or III with associated acetabular fracture

2. **e. A type V fracture consists of a wedge fracture of the medial and lateral plateaux with metaphyseal–diaphyseal discontinuity.**

Tibial plateau fractures usually follow a varus/valgus force with or without axial load. They occur in younger patients following significant trauma, and also in older patients following low-energy injuries (e.g. falls). They are classified according to Schatzker:

I– a lateral split/wedge fracture

II– a lateral split/wedge fracture which is depressed

III– a pure depression fracture, without a split

IV– fracture of the medial plateau

V– bicondylar fracture

VI– associated metaphyseal–diaphyseal discontinuity

Anterior cruciate ligament injuries are more common in type V and VI fractures.

Postgraduate Orthopaedics, ed. Kesavan Sri-Ram. Published by Cambridge University Press.
© Cambridge University Press 2012.

3. **a. On a mortise view, the tibiofibular overlap should normally bc more than 4 mm.**
On a mortise view, the tibiofibular overlap should normally be more than 1 mm.
A Maisonneuve fracture is a proximal fibular fracture associated with a medial malleolar fracture (or disruption of the deltoid ligament), and partial or complete disruption of the syndesmosis. A Dupuytren's fracture-dislocation, described in 1819 by Baron Dupuytren, involves disruption of the medial structures (either a ruptured medial ligament or fracture of the medial malleolus) together with total rupture of the inferior tibiofibular joint and an indirect fracture of the fibula above that syndesmosis. On the mortise view, the talocrual angle is formed by a line drawn parallel to the articular surface of the distal tibia and a line connecting the tips of both malleoli. The angle is normally 8–15°; if there is fibular shortening, this angle will be reduced.

4. **a. Rupture of the extensor pollicis longus (EPL) tendon.**
EPL rupture is seen more commonly with undisplaced distal radial fractures, rather than displaced ones. It is thought that this is due to either a mechanical attrition of the tendon or a local area of ischaemia in the tendon. Repair is not usually possible and treatment is with tendon transfer (EIP to EPL).

5. **e. Interleukin-6 (IL-6).**
Multiple cytokines have been measured in serum. Elevated levels of IL-6 have been associated with the development of MODS.

6. **d. The cortical ring sign is produced by cortex of distal pole of palmar flexed scaphoid.**
A scapholunate distance of more than 2–3 mm as compared to the opposite side is suggestive of scapholunate dissociation. Although Madonna, who is famous for her singing, has a gap between her teeth, it is of course the actor, Terry Thomas, who has given his name to this eponymous sign. On the lateral view, an angle >60–70° suggests scapholunate dissociation.

7. **e. The posterior, transverse portion of medial collateral ligament is the primary stabilizer of the elbow to valgus stress.**
Coronoid fractures are classified as follows: Type I – tip/shear/avulsion; Type II – less than 50% height; Type III – more than 50% height. Based on cadaveric studies, the anterior portion of the medial collateral ligament is the primary stabilizer of the elbow to valgus stress with minimal contribution from the posterior ligament.

8. **a. Enchondral ossification.**
Primary healing (also known as Haversian remodelling) is a direct healing process at the cortex requiring anatomical reduction and rigid stability. Secondary bone healing involves responses in the periosteum and external soft tissues. There are two types; enchondral healing which occurs with non-rigid fixation (such as fracture braces, external fixation, bridge plating, intramedullary nailing); and intramembranous healing which occurs with semi-rigid fixation (such as locked plating in a non-absolute stability construct).

9. **a. Physiotherapy and passive range of motion, 10 days following the injury.**
Immediate physiotherapy and prolonged immobilization are not appropriate in this situation. Although surgical management is an option, a good result can be achieved with non-operative treatment, if the physiotherapy is started within 2 weeks.

10. e. **In a thoracic cord injury, the return of the bulbocavernosus reflex signals the termination of spinal shock.**
The AO classification of spinal fractures is:

  Type A – compression and burst injuries
  Type B – flexion-distraction injuries
  Type C – fracture-dislocation

  When testing myotomes, finger abduction is under the control of the T1 nerve root:
  C5 – shoulder abduction/elbow flexion
  C6 – wrist extension/supination
  C7 – elbow extension/wrist flexion/pronation
  C8 – finger flexion
  T1 – finger abduction

  A Chance fracture is a flexion-distraction injury, which involves two or three columns (anterior may be preserved).

11. c. **Internal fixation of the symphysis pubis and internal fixation of the sacrum.**
Pelvic ring injuries must be assessed for stability, according to the pattern of injury. Classification is either by Tile:

  A – stable
  B – partially stable (rotationally unstable, vertically stable)
  C – unstable (rotationally unstable, vertically unstable)

  or by Young–Burgess:
- Anteroposterior (AP) compression
- Lateral compression
- Vertical shear
- Combined

  This injury described is unstable and requires both anterior and posterior fixation.

12. c. **In the prediction of malunion, the presence or absence of comminution is not an important factor.**
Important factors in predicting early and late instability and radiographic outcome after distal radial fractures include patient age, metaphyseal comminution of the fracture and ulnar variance. Dorsal angulation has not been shown to be significant in the prediction of radiographic outcome for displaced fractures.

13. d. **10% occur in motorcyclists.**
Traumatic scapulothoracic dissociation is a high-energy injury, with associated injury to the brachial plexus and subclavian artery. The mechanism of injury is probably traction caused by a blunt force to the shoulder girdle, commonly seen in motorcyclists (up to 60%). The presence of a complete brachial plexus avulsion is predictive of a poor functional outcome in a patient with scapulothoracic dissociation. Treatment may include vascular repair, plexus exploration and fixation of the commonly associated clavicle fracture to instil stability.

14. e. **Injury to the lateral ascending vessels of the femoral neck.**
Avascular necrosis and collapse of the femoral head following intramedullary nailing of
the femur may be seen if a piriformis fossa entry point is used; this is due to injury to
the lateral ascending cervical artery, which supplies the epiphysis. Therefore, a
piriformis fossa entry point is contraindicated in patients with open physes.

15. c. **It is responsible for bone formation in distraction osteogenesis.**
Intramembranous ossification describes ossification which occurs without a cartilage
model, in comparison to enchondral ossification. Examples of this process include
embryonic flat bone formation (e.g. skull, maxilla, mandible, pelvis, clavicle, subperiosteal
surface of long bone), distraction osteogenesis bone formation, blastema bone (occurs in
children with amputations) and fracture healing with rigid fixation (compression plate).
Hurler's syndrome is a mucopolysaccharidoses (lysosomal storage disease) and
intramembranous ossification in not affected. Cleidocranial dysplasia, however, does
involve defective intramembranous ossification.

16. c. **The highest incidence is seen between the ages 8 and 13.**
The flexion is usually caused by muscle spasm and haemarthrosis. In type III fractures,
the bone fragment may block full extension. The injury is most likely visualized on the
lateral radiograph. Aspiration of a tense haemarthrosis is advised. In a type II
fracture, bony union is possible without reduction manoeuvres.

17. e. **Increase by 16-fold.**
Both the torsional rigidity and bending rigidity of a solid nail are proportional to the radius
to the fourth power. Hence doubling the diameter (and therefore radius) would increase
both these properties 16-fold.

18. e. **Marked osteopaenia.**
The use of locking plates is on the rise. They rely on different mechanical principles compared
to conventional plates. Useful indications include osteoporotic bone, bridging severely
comminuted fractures, plating of fractures where anatomical constraints prevent plating on
the tension side of the bone, and the use of the plate for indirect fracture reduction.

19. c. **Young woman, injured hill-running.**
In general, outcome following operative management of calcaneal fractures relies on the
number of intra-articular fragments and the quality of articular reduction. A number of
factors have been shown to be associated with a poor outcome and they include age >50,
obesity, manual labourers, work insurance cases, smokers, bilateral fractures and vascular
disease. In addition, men appear to do worse with surgery than women.

20. c. **Neurogenic.**
The scenario is explained by a loss of sympathetic outflow, often seen with cervical cord injury.
This gives vasodilatation and decreased venous return with clinical shock. The expected
tachycardia fails to manifest due to unopposed vagal tone, which produces a bradycardia.

21. d. **Arthritis.**
Post-traumatic arthritis is the most common complication following Lisfranc injuries.
The major determinant of a good result is anatomical reduction. Patients with purely

ligamentous injury tend to have outcomes, even with anatomical reduction and screw fixation.

22. d. **It is the 10 cm perforator from the posterior tibial artery, medially which is usually the largest and most reliable for distally based fascio-cutaneous flaps.**
Current management of open fractures has evolved and the involvement of specialist centres is recommended. All wounds do not require immediate exploration. Indications for urgent surgery include gross contamination of the wound, compartment syndrome, a devascularized limb and a multiply injured patient. Otherwise initial surgery (bony and soft tissue) should be performed by senior plastic and orthopaedic surgeons working together on scheduled trauma operating lists within normal working hours and within 24 hours of the injury (unless there is marine, agricultural or sewage contamination).

23. c. **On a serendipity view radiograph, an anterior dislocation would show the affected clavicle above the contralateral clavicle.**
Sternoclavicular dislocations are rare injuries and may be missed if not appropriately imaged. They should not be confused with medial clavicle physeal injuries (this physis fused at around 20–25 years of age). Anterior sternoclavicular dislocations are more common than posterior, and a serendipity view radiograph (beam at 40 cephalic tilt) may help distinguish; in an anterior dislocation, the affected clavicle is above contralateral clavicle, and it is below in a posterior dislocation. The sternoclavicular joint is a diarthrodial saddle joint, with several important ligaments. The posterior capsular ligament is the most important structure for anterior-posterior stability. The anterior sternoclavicular ligament is the primary restraint to superior displacement of medial clavicle. The costoclavicular (rhomboid) ligament has an anterior fasciculus which resists superior rotation and lateral displacement, and a posterior fasciculus which resists inferior rotation and medial displacement. An intra-articular disk ligament prevents medial displacement of clavicle and is a secondary restraint to superior clavicle displacement.

24. c. **Closed reduction in theatre, with reassessment of the vascularity.**
This is a common scenario, and does not always imply a significant arterial injury. It is not appropriate to perform reduction in the emergency department. Instead, a closed reduction, with or without percutaneous K-wiring, should be performed and the vascularity reassessed. Urgent brachial angiography would delay treatment, and primary vascular exploration should not be performed. There is debate as to how urgent reduction should be performed in this scenario; a cold pulseless hand requires urgent treatment.

25. d. **Inadequate closure of the floor of the inguinal canal may lead to an indirect inguinal hernia.**
The anterior ilioinguinal approach allows exposure to the inner surface of the pelvis from the sacroiliac joint to the pubic symphysis, including the anterior and medial surface of acetabulum (and hence anterior column). Three windows are described: lateral (first), middle (second) and medial (third), each allowing exposure of different areas. The corona mortis is a retropubic vascular communication between either the external iliac (or deep epigastric vessels) and the obturator artery, and it may extend over the anterior column in the area of the superior pubic ramus; it is seen in 10–30% of patients and would be seen in the medial window.

26. c. **The pudendal nerve is at risk as it enters the pelvis through the greater sciatic notch.**
The Kocher–Langenbeck approach provides exposure to the posterior wall of and posterior column of acetabulum. It is considered by some as an extension to the posterior approach to the hip and exposes the greater sciatic notch and lesser sciatic notch. The superior gluteal artery and nerve are at risk of injury here and must be protected. The pudendal nerve is at risk, but it exits the pelvis via the greater sciatic notch and re-enters via the lesser sciatic notch.

27. b. **Increasing the distance between the rods and the bone.**
The principle factor which contributes to external fixator stability is reduction of the fracture. Other factors which would increase the stability are:

Increased pin diameter
Increased number of pins
Decreased bone to rod distance
Pins placed in different planes
Increased size or stacking rods
Rods in different planes
Increased spacing between pins

28. d. **Posterior column and posterior hemitransverse.**
The Judet and Letournel classification describe 10 fracture patterns:

Simple fractures

- posterior wall
- posterior column
- anterior wall
- anterior column
- transverse

Complex/associated fracture

- both columns
- posterior wall and transverse
- T-shaped fracture
- anterior column and posterior hemitransverse
- posterior wall and posterior column

29. c. **Fracture at the metaphyseal–diaphyseal junction of the fifth metatarsal at the level of the fourth–fifth intermetatarsal articulation.**
Fractures of the base of the fifth metatarsal are common. They are classified into zones according to location:

Zone 1 – Proximal metaphyseal fracture of the fifth metatarsal at the level of the tarsometatarsal joint
Zone 2 – Fracture at the metaphyseal–diaphyseal junction of the fifth metatarsal at the level of the fourth–fifth intermetatarsal articulation
Zone 3 – Fracture at the proximal diaphysis of the fifth metatarsal distal to the level of the fourth–fifth intermetatarsal articulation

The zone 2 injury is also known as a Jones fracture, after Sir Robert Jones.

30. b. **Associated radial nerve palsy**.

Humeral shaft fractures are common, and most can be treated in a functional brace, assuming there is <20° anterior angulation, <30° varus/valgus angulation and <3 cm shortening. Contraindications to functional bracing include a severe soft tissue injury or bone loss, an uncooperative patient, polytrauma (especially ipsilateral injuries), associated brachial plexus injury and fractures in the proximal one-third of the humerus. Radial nerve palsy alone is not a contraindication.

EMQs

1. 1. **f. 2.5 mm**. 2. **k. 3.5 mm**. 3. **h. 2.8 mm**.

Although we commonly ask for the 'gold' or 'silver' drill, it is important to be aware of the various drill, tap and screw sizes available on the standard fracture fixation sets. These are summarized:

Small fragment set

Screw type	Cortical	Cortical	Cancellous	Locking	Locking
Thread diameter	2.7 mm	3.5 mm	4.0 mm	2.7 mm	3.5 mm
Drill bit size	2.0 mm	2.5 mm	2.5 mm	2.0 mm	2.8 mm
Tap size	2.7 mm	3.5 mm	4.0 mm	Self tap	Self tap

Large fragment set

Screw type	Cortical	Cortical	Cancellous	Locking	Locking
Thread diameter	4.5 mm	5.5 mm	6.5 mm	4.0 mm	5.0 mm
Drill bit size	3.2 mm	4.0 mm	3.2 mm	3.2 mm	4.3 mm
Tap size	4.5 mm	5.5 mm	6.5 mm	Self tap	Self tap

2. 1. **g. 9**. 2. **c. B3**. 3. **d. 2**.

Mirel's score is used as a predictor of fracture in pathological lesions. A score greater than 7 suggests a high risk:

Score	1	2	3
Site	Upper limb	Lower limb	Peri-trochanteric
Pain	Mild	Moderate	Functional
Lesion	Blastic	Mixed	Lytic
Size	<1/3	1/3–2/3	>2/3

The 'Vancouver' classification is used for periprosthetic fractures around hip implants as follows:

Type A – trochanteric region
Type B1 – around or just below a well-fixed stem
Type B2 – around or just below a loose stem, with good proximal bone stock
Type B3 – around or just below a loose stem, with poor proximal bone stock
Type C – well below the prosthesis

The Oestern and Tscherne classification for soft tissue injury in closed fractures is:

Grade 0 – minimal soft tissue injury; simple fracture pattern
Grade I – superficial abrasion; mild fracture pattern
Grade II – deep abrasion; skin or muscle contusion; severe fracture pattern
Grade III – extensive contusion or crush injury; muscle damage; compartment syndrome; subcutaneous avulsion

3. 1. **h. Jefferson's fracture**. 2. **b. Pseudosubluxation**. 3. **f. Unilateral facet dislocation**.
A Jefferson's fracture is classically described as a four-part burst fracture of the atlas,
with combined anterior and posterior arch fractures. It may also be caused by
hyperextension. Pseudosubluxation is normal in children up to the age of 8 years and is
due to increased ligamentous laxity and a more horizontal nature of facet joint. It
occurs between C2 and C3 or between C3 and C4. The 'bow tie' sign refers to the
two lateral masses of dislocated vertebrae overlapping partially on lateral radiograph,
in a unilateral facet dislocation.

4. 1. **b. Monteggia fracture**. 2. **d. Rolando fracture**. 3. **g. Essex-Lopresti injury**.
Eponymous names for fractures are common and continue to be used. Monteggia fractures
(proximal ulna fracture and associated radial head dislocation are classified by Bado).
A Rolando fracture is a Y- or T-shaped intra-articular fracture of the base of the thumb
metacarpal. The Essex-Lopresti injury is a radial head fracture, with interosseous membrane
disruption and subluxation or dislocation of the distal radioulnar joint.

5. 1. **g. Ilioischial line**. 2. **a. Shenton's line**. 3. **d. Hilgenreiner's line**.
A number of lines appear on a pelvis radiograph, and knowledge of them is important, as
disruption of the lines usually implies abnormality. Shenton's line is a curvilinear line
along the inferior margin of the superior pubic ramus which continues along the inferior
border of the femoral neck. Nelaton's line is not a radiographic line, but instead is a line
from the anterior superior iliac spine to the tuberosity of the ischium. Klein's line is a line
drawn along the superior border of the femoral neck. Hilgenreiner's line is a line drawn
between the two tri-radiate cartilages. Trethowan's line does not exist, although
Trethowan's sign is positive when Klein's line does not pass through the femoral head.
Perkin's line is a line drawn perpendicular to Hilgenreiner's line, intersecting the
lateralmost aspect of the acetabular roof. Ilioischial line demarcates the medial border of
the posterior column of the acetabulum. Iliopectineal line demarcates the anterior
column of the acetabulum. Iliopubic line is an alternative name for the iliopectineal line.
The Northern line does not appear on a pelvis!

6. 1. **b. Central cord syndrome**. 2. **a. Brown-Séquard syndrome**. 3. **i. None of the
above**.
The Brown-Séquard syndrome occurs with a cord hemitransection and carries the best
prognosis. It is characterized by a motor deficit and numbness to touch and vibration on
the same side of the spinal injury and loss of pain and temperature sensation on the
opposite side. Central cord syndrome carries a less favourable prognosis with only 10–15%
of patients demonstrating functional recovery.

7. 1. **d. Anterior interosseous nerve**. 2. **c. Median nerve**. 3. **i. Musculocutaneous nerve**.
The inability to flex at the index finger distal interphalangeal joint suggests the interosseous
nerve is injured, and the ability to flex at the ring finger distal interphalangeal joint
confirms that the median nerve is intact. The Camitz transfer involves transferring palmaris
longus to abductor pollicis brevis, to restore thumb function. Therefore in this case the
median nerve (and hence recurrent motor branch) is not functioning. Numbness over the
lateral aspect of the forearm implies injury to the musculocutaneous nerve, which
terminates as the lateral cutaneous nerve of the forearm.

8. 1. **c. 4**. 2. **d. 5**. 3. **g. 10**.

The Mangled Extremity Severity Score (MESS) is useful in determining the prognosis of an injured limb. The scoring is as follows:

Skeletal/soft tissue injury

> 1– Low energy (stab; simple fracture; pistol gunshot wound)
> 2– Medium energy (open or multiple fractures, dislocation)
> 3– High energy (high speed road traffic accident or rifle gunshot wound)
> 4– Very high energy (high-speed trauma + gross contamination)

Limb ischaemia (score doubled if ischaemia time >6 hours)

> 1– Pulse reduced or absent but perfusion normal
> 2– Pulseless; paraesthesia, diminished capillary refill
> 3– Cool, paralyzed, insensate, numb

Shock

> 0– Systolic blood pressure (BP) always >90 mmHg
> 1– Hypotensive transiently
> 2– Persistent hypotension

Age

> 0– <30 years
> 1– 30–50 years
> 2– >50 years

A MESS Score >7 suggests a poor limb viability prognosis.

9. 1. **l. D and E**. 2. **h. Capitellum fracture**. 3. **j. Elbow dislocation**.

A terrible triad injury is classically described as a posterolateral dislocation with associated radial head and coronoid fractures. Fractures of the capitellum are classified with eponymous terms: Type 1 (Hahn–Steinthal) consists of a large fragment of cancellous bone of the articular surface of the capitellum and may include a portion of the trochlea, typically the lateral third; type 2 (Kocher–Lorenz) is a cartilaginous articular fracture of the capitellum and may include a small fragment of subchondral bone typically described as 'uncapping' of the capitellum; type 3 (Broberg and Morrey) is a comminuted capitellar fracture. In an adult, an elbow dislocation is most likely to be associated with vascular injury (as opposed to a supracondylar fracture in a child).

10. 1. **d. Young–Burgess**. 2. **e. Damschen**. 3. **g. Mason**.

Numerous classifications are used in trauma and orthopaedics and include Mayfield (perilunate dislocation), Tile (pelvis injury), Garden (neck of femur fracture), Young–Burgess (pelvis injury), Damschen (scapulothoracic dissociation), Essex-Lopresti (calcaneal fractures), Mason (radial head fractures), AO (generic fracture classification), Bado (Monteggia fracture-dislocation), Frykman (distal radial fractures), Gustillo (open fractures).

11. 1. **g. Unreamed intramedullary nailing with static interlocking**. 2. **d. Retrograde flexible intramedullary nailing**. 3. **j. Observation**.

Closed diaphyseal femoral fractures in adults are best treated with reamed intramedullary nailing with static interlocking. This is because reaming allows placement of a larger, stronger implant and offers better healing rates than unreamed nailing. Static locking should ensure that there is maintenance of reduction. In children less than 11 and of normal weight, retrograde flexible intramedullary nailing for femoral shaft fractures have shown many good to excellent results. Following proximal tibial metaphyseal fractures in children, a late genu valgum deformity can develop due to asymmetric growth of the proximal tibia (Cozen's). These children should be treated with observation because the deformity is likely to remodel.

12. 1. **d. 4**. 2. **j. 10**. 3. **c. 3**.
It is important to be aware of the number of osteofascial compartments in various regions of the body, particularly with respect to surgical decompression of compartment syndrome. The leg has 4 compartments (anterior, lateral, superficial posterior and deep posterior). The hand has 10 compartments (dorsal interossei × 4, palmar interossei × 3, adductor pollicis, thenar and hypothenar). The forearm has 3 compartments (superficial flexor, deep flexor and extensor).

13. 1. **a. Pellegrini–Stieda**. 2. **b. Hoffa**. 3. **c. Segond**.
Pellegrini–Stieda lesion refers to mineralization near to the medial femoral epicondyle, where the medial collateral attaches. It follows injury to the ligament and can result in persistent pain known as Pellegrini–Stieda syndrome. A coronal plane fracture of the femoral condyle is termed a Hoffa's fracture. A Segond injury refers to the lateral tibial plateau capsule avulsion injury, which corresponds to an anterior cruciate ligament injury.

14. 1. **g. Smith–Petersen**. 2. **c. Henry's**. 3. **g. Smith–Petersen**.
The Smith–Peterson (anterior) approach to the hip takes place between sartorius (femoral nerve) and tensor fascia lata (superior gluteal nerve) superficially, and between rectus femoris (femoral nerve) and gluteus medius (superior gluteal nerve) deep. During superficial dissection, the ascending branch of the lateral femoral circumflex artery will be encountered, as it crosses the gap between sartorius and tensor fascia lata; it should be ligated. Henry's approach involves an internervous plane between the radial and median nerves, i.e. between brachioradialis (radial nerve) and pronator teres proximally and flexor carpi radialis distally (both median nerve).

15. 1. **i. Basilar skull fracture**. 2. **c. Epidural haemorrhage**. 3. **d. Subdural haemorrhage**.
The Battle's sign is bruising over the mastoid process, as a result of extravasation of blood along the path of the posterior auricular artery and indicates a basilar skull fracture. Other clinical signs include haemotympanum, and cerebrospinal fluid rhinorrhoea and otorrhoea. Bleeding from the middle meningeal artery gives rise to an epidural haematoma, which, on CT scan, appears as a convex-shaped lesion in the epidural space. Bleeding from the bridging veins gives rise to a subdural haematoma, which appears as a crescent-shaped lesion in the subdural space.

Selected references

Buckley R, Tough S, McCormack R *et al.* Operative compared with nonoperative treatment of displaced intra-articular calcaneal fractures: a prospective, randomized, controlled multicenter trial. *J Bone Joint Surg Am* 2002; **84**(10): 1733–44.

Cozen L. Knock-knee deformity in children: congenital and acquired. *Clin Orthop* 1990; **258**: 191–203.

Ebraheim NA, An HS, Jackson WT *et al.* Scapulothoracic dissociation. *J Bone Joint Surg Am* 1988; **70**(3): 428–32.

Giannoudis PV, Smith RM, Banks RE *et al.* Stimulation of inflammatory markers after blunt trauma. *Br J Surg* 1998; **85**(7): 986–90.

Hotchkiss RN, Weiland AJ. Valgus stability of the elbow. *J Orthop Res* 1987; **5**(3): 372–7.

Koval KJ, Gallagher MA, Marsicano JG *et al.* Functional outcome after minimally displaced fractures of the proximal part of the humerus. *J Bone Joint Surg Am* 1997; **79**(2): 203–7.

Kuo RS, Tejwani NC, Digiovanni CW *et al.* Outcome after open reduction and internal fixation of Lisfranc joint injuries. *J Bone Joint Surg Am* 2000; **82**(11): 1609–18.

Letts M, Jarvis J, Lawton L, Davidson D. Complications of rigid intramedullary rodding of femoral shaft fractures in children. *J Trauma* 2002; **52**(3): 504–16.

Mackenney PJ, McQueen MM, Elton R. Prediction of instability in distal radial fractures. *J Bone Joint Surg Am* 2006; **88**(9): 1944–51.

Meyers MH, McKeever FM. Fracture of the intercondylar eminence of the tibia. *J Bone Joint Surg Am* 1959; **41**(2): 209–22.

Omid R, Choi PD, Skaggs DL. Supracondylar humeral fractures in children. *J Bone Joint Surg Am* 2008; **90**(5): 1121–32.

Pipkin G. Treatment of grade IV fracture-dislocation of the hip. *J Bone Joint Surg Am* 1957; **39**(5): 1027–42.

Schatzker J, Tile M. *The Rationale of Operative Fracture Care.* 3rd edn. New York, Springer, 2005.

The Working Group (BOA/BAPRAS). *Standards for the Management of Open Fractures of the Lower Limb. A Short Guide.* 2009.

Thompson VP, Epstein HC. Traumatic dislocation of the hip: a survey of two hundred and four cases covering a period of twenty-one years. *J Bone Joint Surg Am* **195**; 33: 746–78.

Tile M, Helfet D, Kellam J. *Fractures of the Pelvis and Acetabulum.* 3rd edn. Philadelphia, Lippincott Williams and Wilkins, 2003.

Zelle BA, Pape HC, Gerich TG *et al.* Functional outcome following scapulothoracic dissociation. *J Bone Joint Surg Am* 2004; **86**(1): 2–8.

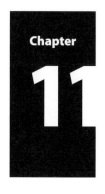

Chapter

1

Basic science: Questions

Ben Rudge and John A. Skinner

MCQs

1. **Which of the following definitions with reference to screening programmes is correct?**
   a. Prevalence is the rate of occurrence of new disease within a disease-free population.
   b. Sensitivity is the ability of a screening test to exclude false negatives.
   c. Specificity is the ability of a test to pick up all the cases of a disease.
   d. Positive predictive value is calculated by dividing all the positive test results by all the negative results.
   e. Incidence is the frequency of a disease at any given time.

2. **Which of the following correctly describes the pattern of inheritance for the corresponding condition?**
   a. Achondroplasia – autosomal Recessive.
   b. Osteogenesis imperfecta type 1 – autosomal Recessive.
   c. Sickle cell anaemia – autosomal Recessive.
   d. Hypophosphataemic rickets – X-linked Recessive.
   e. Duchenne's muscular dystrophy – X-linked Dominant.

3. **Which of the following statements regarding physes is incorrect?**
   a. The strength in each layer of the physis is related to the proportion of extracellular matrix present.
   b. The hypertrophic layer is the weakest layer of the physis.
   c. Approximately 75% of the growth of the radius occurs at its distal end.
   d. The hip, knee, shoulder and elbow have intra-articular physes that can account for progression of metaphyseal osteomyelitis to septic arthritis.
   e. The apophysis of the ileum closes from lateral to medial.

4. **Which of the following descriptions of antibiotic mechanism of action is incorrect?**
   a. Ciprofloxacin inhibits DNA gyrase.
   b. Aminoglycosides exert their bactericidal effect by binding to the 30S subunit.
   c. Rifampicin inhibits DNA polymerase.
   d. Erythromycin acts by binding to the 30S subunit.
   e. Vancomycin inhibits cell membrane synthesis.

Postgraduate Orthopaedics, ed. Kesavan Sri-Ram. Published by Cambridge University Press.
© Cambridge University Press 2012.

5. **Which of the following bacterial classifications is incorrect?**
   a. *Clostridium perfringens* is a Gram-positive bacillus.
   b. *Eikenella corrodens* is a Gram-negative bacillus.
   c. *Staphylococcus epidermidis* is a Gram-positive coccus.
   d. *Pseudomonas* is a Gram-negative coccus.
   e. E. coli is a Gram-negative bacillus.

6. **Which of the following statements is incorrect with regards to dual-energy X-ray absorptiometry (DEXA) scanning?**
   a. DEXA scans assess bone mineral density.
   b. Cortical and cancellous bone densities are indistinguishable on DEXA scans of the proximal femur.
   c. Vertebral fractures may give rise to false low density values.
   d. Osteoporosis is defined by a T-score lower than –2.5.
   e. A low Z-score indicates non age related bone loss.

7. **A biopsy taken from an Achilles tendon, 5 days after rupture treated in plaster, would show a predominance of which collagen subtype?**
   a. I.
   b. II.
   c. III.
   d. IV.
   e. X.

8. **Which of the following incorrectly describes changes in articular cartilage?**
   a. Water content increases in osteoarthritis.
   b. Water content decreases as part of ageing.
   c. Young's modulus of elasticity increases in ageing.
   d. Proteoglycan degradation increases in osteoarthritis.
   e. Chondrocyte number increases in ageing.

9. **With reference to a cross section of the spinal cord, which of the following descriptions is incorrect?**
   a. Pain and temperature sensation is transmitted via the lateral spinothalamic tracts.
   b. Light touch is transmitted in the anterior spinothalamic tract.
   c. Deep touch is transmitted in the dorsal columns.
   d. Proprioception is transmitted in the dorsal columns.
   e. Vibration is transmitted in the anterior corticospinal tract.

10. **To which of the following groups do most of the bone morphogenetic proteins belong?**
    a. Platelet-derived growth factors.
    b. Fibroblast growth factors.
    c. Transforming growth factors.
    d. Vascular endothelial-derived growth factor.
    e. Insulin-like growth factors.

11. **Which of the following statements regarding bone cell biology is incorrect?**
    a. Parathyroid hormone (PTH) acts directly on osteoclasts to stimulate bone resorption via carbonic anhydrase.
    b. Calcitonin acts directly on osteoclasts to inhibit bone resorption.
    c. Interleukin-1 is a potent stimulator of osteoclastic bone resorption.
    d. Osteoblasts have receptors for PTH, 1,25 dihydroxy vitamin D, glucocorticoids, prostaglandins and oestrogen.
    e. Osteocytes are former osteoblasts.

12. **Which is the correct formula for calcium hydroxyapatite?**
    a. $Ca_2 (PO_4)_6 (OH)_2$.
    b. $Ca_{10} (PO_4)_2 (OH)_{10}$.
    c. $Ca_{10} (PO_4)_6 (OH)_2$.
    d. $CaPO_4OH_2$.
    e. $Ca_2 (PO_4)_{10} (OH)_6$.

13. **Which of the following is not a prerequisite of gait?**
    a. Foot prepositioning.
    b. Stability in stance.
    c. Adequate stride length.
    d. Conservation of energy.
    e. Clearance in swing phase.

14. **Which of the following statements regarding energy requirements following amputations is incorrect?**
    a. A below knee amputee (BKA) requires a 25% increase in energy expenditure for ambulation.
    b. A transfemoral amputee requires a 65% increase in energy expenditure for ambulation.
    c. The increase in metabolic cost of amputation is inversely proportional to the length of the residium.
    d. Wheelchair use requires 5% increase in energy expenditure.
    e. A bilateral above knee amputee (AKA) requires 80% increase in energy expenditure for ambulation.

15. **Which of the following statements regarding polymethylmethacrylate (PMMA) cement is incorrect?**
    a. It is strongest in compression.
    b. It has poor tensile strength.
    c. It exhibits a high Young's modulus.
    d. It exhibits viscoelastic properties.
    e. It has very poor adhesive properties.

16. **According to Mirels' scoring system a patient with a very large, metastatic, pertrochanteric, painless lytic lesion would have a score of?**
    a. 4.
    b. 6.
    c. 8.

d. 10.

e. 12.

17. **Which of the following statements regarding muscle activity in the three rockers of stance phase is correct?**
    a. During the first rocker, concentric contraction of tibialis anterior prevents foot-slap.
    b. Eccentric contraction of the ankle dorsiflexors occurs during the second rocker.
    c. Eccentric contraction of the ankle plantarflexors occurs during the first rocker.
    d. Concentric contraction of tibialis anterior occurs during the third rocker.
    e. Eccentric contraction of gastro-soleus occurs during the second rocker.

18. **Which of the following lists of materials is correctly ordered with respect to their Young's modulus of elasticity from high to low?**
    a. Titanium, stainless steel, cobalt chrome, cortical bone, polymethylmethacrylate (PMMA) cement, ultra-high-molecular-weight polyethylene (UHWMPE).
    b. Cobalt chrome, stainless steel, titanium, cortical bone, PMMA cement, UHWMPE.
    c. Stainless steel, cobalt chrome, titanium, cortical bone, PMMA cement, UHWMPE.
    d. Cortical bone, cancellous bone, PMMA cement, UHWMPE, tendon, cartilage.
    e. Titanium, cortical bone, UHWMPE, PMMA cement, cancellous bone, tendon.

19. **Which of the following is not a recognized World Health Organization (WHO) requirement for a screening test?**
    a. The treatment for the disease being screened for is accepted and effective.
    b. The natural history of the condition is known.
    c. The screening programme should be cost effective.
    d. The test is acceptable to the patient.
    e. The disease should be one in which late treatment is as effective as early treatment.

20. **Which of the following statements concerning limb embryology is false?**
    a. The apical ectodermal ridge forms at about 4 weeks in utero.
    b. The zone of proliferating activity controls limb growth in a proximal to distal direction.
    c. The limb buds develop between 4 and 6 weeks in utero.
    d. The lower limb buds rotate internally after formation.
    e. Primary ossification centres form at approximately 8 weeks in utero.

21. **As a cemented femoral component of a total hip arthroplasty fails by cantilever bending a plain anteroposterior (AP) pelvic radiograph will reveal?**
    a. Radiolucent lines in Gruen zones 1 to 7 inclusive.
    b. Cement mantle fracture in Gruen zones 2 and 6.
    c. Radiolucent lines in Gruen zones 4 and 5.
    d. Lateral migration of the distal stem tip.
    e. Radiolucent lines in Gruen zones 1, 2, 6 and 7.

22. **Which of the following tumours is the most likely diagnosis in a 13-year-old boy presenting with a mid-femoral lesion with a large associated soft tissue swelling?**
    a. Chondrosarcoma.
    b. Osteosarcoma.

   c. Ewing's sarcoma.
   d. Giant cell tumour.
   e. Fibrous dysplasia.

23. **The posterior interosseus nerve can be compressed in all of the following sites except?**
   a. The leash of Henry.
   b. The arcade of Frohse.
   c. The distal margin of the supinator muscle.
   d. Extensor carpi radialis brevis (ECRB).
   e. The ligament of Struthers.

24. **All of the following nerves have a contribution from the fifth cervical nerve except?**
   a. The lateral pectoral nerve.
   b. The axillary nerve.
   c. The upper subscapular nerve.
   d. The thoracodorsal nerve.
   e. The radial nerve.

25. **A muscle contraction during which tension is constant throughout the range of motion but muscle length changes is referred to as?**
   a. Isometric.
   b. Plyometric.
   c. Isokinetic.
   d. Closed chain.
   e. Isotonic.

26. **In the microstructure of muscle which of the following represents the boundary between two sarcomeres?**
   a. I band.
   b. A band.
   c. M line.
   d. Z disc.
   e. H band.

27. **Which of the following terms describes how health services are held accountable for the safety, quality and effectiveness of clinical care delivered to patients?**
   a. Appraisal.
   b. Revalidation.
   c. Licensing.
   d. Clinical effectiveness.
   e. Clinical governance.

28. **With regards to bone grafting, the term osteoconductive refers to?**
   a. The content of living cells which can differentiate into bone-producing cells.
   b. The biological stimulus provided by the graft.
   c. The graft's three-dimensional scaffold for bone ingrowth.
   d. The inclusion of bone morphogenetic proteins (BMPs).
   e. The immunogenic potential of the graft.

29. **With reference to biomaterials, brittleness refers to?**
    a. A material that can undergo extensive plastic deformation prior to failure.
    b. A surface property of the material.
    c. A material's deflection for a given load.
    d. A material that has an elastic limit that approximates its fracture point.
    e. The maximum amount of stress the material can withstand before failing.

30. **The pull-out strength of a cortical screw can be increased by?**
    a. Changing to a larger core diameter.
    b. Changing to a smaller outer diameter.
    c. The addition of a self-tapping tip.
    d. Changing to a finer pitch.
    e. Adding a locking thread to the head.

EMQs

1. **Types of study**
   a. Case study
   b. Case series
   c. Case–control study
   d. Cross-sectional study
   e. Cohort study
   f. Randomized controlled trial
   g. Equivalence study
   h. Sequential analysis
   i. Systematic review
   j. Meta-analysis

Which of the options above is best described in each of the following statements? Each option may be used once, more than once or not at all.
   1. Two groups of patients are followed over time to compare outcomes.
   2. Reporting on the outcome of a group of patients.
   3. Having appraised a number of relevant papers, a common estimate is reported with confidence intervals.

2. **Definitions in statistics**
   a. Variance
   b. Standard deviation
   c. Standard error of the mean
   d. Confidence interval
   e. Null hypothesis
   f. P value
   g. Type 1 (alpha) error
   h. Type 2 (beta) error
   i. Power

Which of the options above is best described in each of the following statements? Each option may be used once, more than once or not at all.
   1. This is determined by taking the square root of the variance.
   2. This is a false-negative result – i.e. the null hypothesis is incorrectly accepted.
   3. This is taken as $1 -$ type 2 error.

3. **Corrosion**
   a. Passivation
   b. Uniform attack
   c. Galvanic
   d. Crevice
   e. Fretting
   f. Pitting
   g. Intergranular
   h. Inclusion
   i. Fatigue

Which of the options above is best described in each of the following statements?
Each option may be used once, more than once or not at all.
1. This is when two dissimilar metals become electrically coupled.
2. This describes a combination of wear and crevice corrosion.
3. This process is characterized by an area of oxygen depletion preventing passivation.

4. **Disorders of the physis**
   a. Reserve zone
   b. Proliferative zone
   c. Maturation zone
   d. Degenerative zone
   e. Zone of provisional calcification
   f. Primary spongiosa
   g. Secondary spongiosa

Which of the options above is best described in each of the following statements?
Each option may be used once, more than once or not at all.
1. The layer affected in achondroplasia.
2. The layer affected in pseudoachondroplasia.
3. The layer affected in Gaucher's disease.

5. **Neurophysiology tests**
   a. Latency
   b. Velocity
   c. Amplitude
   d. Sensory nerve action potentials (SNAP)
   e. Compound nerve action potentials (CNAP)
   f. Somatosensory-evoked potentials (SSEP)
   g. H reflex
   h. F response

Which of the options above is best described in each of the following statements?
Each option may be used once, more than once or not at all.
1. A measure of the antidromic conduction of an impulse from a peripheral nerve to the anterior horn cell along with its reflex orthodromic conduction to the muscle.
2. This is measured in spinal cord monitoring intraoperatively, by stimulating peripheral nerves and recording the stimulus from the scalp.
3. This is a measure of the time between onset of stimulus and response.

6. **Lubrication**
   a. Boundary
   b. Fluid film
   c. Hydrodynamic
   d. Elastohydrodynamic
   e. Microelastohydrodynamic
   f. Squeeze film
   g. Weeping
   h. Boosted

Which of the options above is best described in each of the following statements? Each option may be used once, more than once or not at all.

1. This occurs when bearing surfaces approach each other without relative sliding motion, i.e. in the hip joint at heel-strike.
2. This occurs as water moves into cartilage leaving an increased concentration of hyaluronic acid–protein complexes for lubrication.
3. This predominates in metal on polyethylene hip arthroplasty articulations.

7. **Material properties**
   a. Viscoelastic
   b. Plastic
   c. Ductile
   d. Anisotropic
   e. Isotropic
   f. Hardness
   g. Toughness
   h. Brittle
   i. Creep
   j. Stress relaxation
   k. Hysteresis

Which of the options above is best described in each of the following statements? Each option may be used once, more than once or not at all.

1. This is represented by the area under the stress–strain curve.
2. This can be defined as time-dependent deformation in response to a constant load.
3. This describes a material with a yield point that is almost equivalent to its ultimate tensile stress.

8. **Pathogens**
   a. *Pasteurella multocida*
   b. *Streptococcus viridans*
   c. Group A streptococcus
   d. *Clostridium perfringens*
   e. *Mycobacterium marinarum*
   f. *Streptococcus pyogenes*
   g. *Clostridium difficile*
   h. *Vibrio vulnificus*

Which of the options above is best described in each of the following statements? Each option may be used once, more than once or not at all.

1. A diabetic man presents to the casualty department with septic shock 24 hours after spending the day fly-fishing.
2. A bare-knuckle prize-fighter presents 2 days after a bout with a swollen hand and a weeping wound over his middle finger metacarpophalangeal joint.
3. A 64-year-old lady presents having been bitten by a greyhound the previous day whilst out running.

9. **Metabolic bone diseases**
   a. Primary hyperparathyroidism
   b. Hyperthyroidism
   c. Malignancy with bone metastases
   d. Pseudohypoparathyroidism
   e. Vitamin D deficiency
   f. Renal osteodystrophy
   g. Paget's disease
   h. Hypophosphatasia
   i. Hypophosphataemic rickets

Which of the options above is best described in each of the following statements?
Each option may be used once, more than once or not at all.
   1. An autosomal recessive disorder with increased urinary phosphoethanolamine.
   2. The test results in this include a raised alkaline phosphatase and urine hydroxyproline.
   3. The test results in this include a markedly raised serum phosphorous and parathyroid hormone with radiographs revealing a 'rugger-jersey' spine.

10. **Genetic defects**
   a. Achondroplasia
   b. Duchenne's muscular dystrophy
   c. Osteogenesis imperfecta
   d. Marfan's
   e. Multiple hereditory exostoses
   f. Pseudoachondroplasia
   g. Multiple epiphyseal dysplasia
   h. Hypophosphataemic rickets
   i. Diastrophic dysplasia

Which of the options above is best described in each of the following statements?
Each option may be used once, more than once or not at all.
   1. A condition associated with a defect in fibrillin.
   2. A condition associated with a defect in the EXT1/EXT2 genes.
   3. A condition associated with a defect in dystrophin.

11. **Statistical tests**
   a. Student's t-test
   b. ANOVA
   c. Chi-squared test
   d. Pearson correlation
   e. Spearman correlation
   f. Mann–Whitney U test
   g. Kruskal–Wallis test
   h. Bonferonni correction
   i. Kaplan–Meier method

Which of the options above is best described in each of the following statements?
Each option may be used once, more than once or not at all.

1. A test performed to reduce the risk of a type 1 error when performing multiple tests.
2. A parametric test used to compare a pair of observations on a single subject.
3. This quantifies the association between two variables from parametric data.

12. **Implant manufacture**
    a. Direct compression moulding
    b. Sintering
    c. Ram extrusion
    d. Plasma spraying
    e. Shot blasting
    f. Annealing
    g. Cold working

Which of the options above is best described in each of the following statements?
Each option may be used once, more than once or not at all.
1. The method by which hydroxyapatite coating is applied to metallic implants.
2. Polyethylene undergoes this process after high dose gamma irradiation, the purpose being to remove free radicals.
3. This process is used in the manufacture of ceramics from a powder substrate.

13. **Definitions in mechanics**
    a. Equilibrium
    b. Moment
    c. Ground reaction force
    d. Joint reaction force
    e. Weight
    f. Mass
    g. Friction
    h. Inertia
    i. Force

Which of the options above is best described in each of the following statements?
Each option may be used once, more than once or not at all.
1. A quantity of heaviness that depends on the local gravitational field.
2. A force resisting the relative motion of solid surfaces in contact.
3. This equates to Newton's First Law.

14. **The brachial plexus**
    a. Lateral cord
    b. Posterior cord
    c. Anterior cord
    d. Medial cord
    e. Superior (upper) trunk
    f. Middle trunk
    g. Inferior (lower) trunk
    h. Roots

Select the site of origin from the options above that best fits the nerves named below. Each option may be used once, more than once or not at all.

1. The site of origin of the suprascapular nerve.
2. The site of origin of the thoracodorsal nerve.
3. The site of origin of the lower subscapular nerve.

15. **Examination of the lower limb**
   a. Thomas'
   b. Faber
   c. Ely's
   d. Barlow's
   e. Ortolani's
   f. Galleazi's
   g. Trendelenburg
   h. Fadir

Which of the options above is best described in each of the following statements? Each option may be used once, more than once or not at all.

1. This test detects a tight rectus femoris by flexing the knee while prone.
2. This test involves attempting to reduce a dislocated hip.
3. A positive test suggests either developmental dysplasia of the hip or a leg length discrepancy.

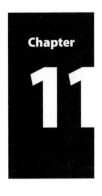

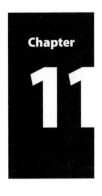

Chapter

11

Basic science: Answers

Ben Rudge and John A. Skinner

MCQs

1. b. Sensitivity is the ability of a screening test to exclude false negatives.
Prevalence is defined as the frequency of a disease at a given time, i.e. of all the patients at risk of having the disease how many actually have it now. Incidence is the rate of occurrence of new disease within a disease-free population, i.e. how frequently does another one come up. Specificity is the ability of a test to exclude a disease, i.e. exclude false positives. Sensitivity is the ability of a screening test to exclude false negatives. Positive predictive value is the probability that a subject with a positive test result actually has the disease. It is found by dividing all true positive test results by the total number of positive test results.

2. c. Sickle cell anaemia – autosomal Recessive.
As a very general rule of thumb autosomal dominant disorders cause structural defects whereas autosomal recessive defects are physiological. In orthopaedics, X-linked hypophosphataemic rickets is the only X-linked dominant condition to be aware of.

3. d. The hip, knee, shoulder and elbow have intra-articular physes that can account for progression of metaphyseal osteomyelitis to septic arthritis.
The joints with intra-articlular physes are the shoulder (humerus), elbow (radial head), hip (proximal femur) and ankle (lateral malleolus).

4. d. Erythromycin acts by binding to the 30S subunit.
Erythromycin binds to the 50S subunit. This can be easily remembered, i.e. *amino*glycosides bind to the 30S subunit whereas the *macro*lides bind to the 50S subunit.

5. d. *Pseudomonas* is a Gram-negative coccus.
Pseudomonas is a Gram-negative bacillus. Common bacteria include:

Gram-positive coccus	Gram-negative coccus	Gram-positive bacillus	Gram-negative bacillus
Staphylococcus aureus	*Neisseria gonorrhoea*	*Clostridia* (*tetani, perfringens, difficile*)	*Pseudomonas aeruginosa*
Enterococcus	*Neisseria meningitides*	*Listeria monocytogenes*	*Eikenella corrodens*

Postgraduate Orthopaedics, ed. Kesavan Sri-Ram. Published by Cambridge University Press.
© Cambridge University Press 2012.

Gram-positive coccus	Gram-negative coccus	Gram-positive bacillus	Gram-negative bacillus
Steptococcus		Actinomyces	Escherichia coli
		Coryneform	Salmonella typhi
		Diphtheroids	Klebsiella pneumoniae
			Helicobacter pylori

6. c. **Vertebral fractures may give rise to false low density values.**
DEXA scanning is used to assess bone mineral density, in particular to diagnose osteoporosis. Vertebral fractures may give rise to falsely elevated bone density values.

7. c. **III.**
There are several collagen types, including:

Type I collagen is the predominant form in bone and fibrocartilage
Type II collagen is found in articular cartilage
Type III collagen is produced in the proliferative phase of tendon and ligament healing
Type IV collagen forms the bases of cell basement membranes
Type X collagen is found in mineralizing cartilage in endochondral ossification

8. e. **Chondrocyte number increases in ageing.**
Chondrocyte numbers decrease in ageing cartilage. The others are all true:

	Osteoarthritis	Ageing
Water content	Increases	Decreases
Proteoglycan degradation	Increases	Decreases
Chondrocyte number	Decreases	Decreases
Young's modulus of elasticity	Decreases	Increases

9. e. **Vibration is transmitted in the anterior corticospinal tract.**
Vibration is also transmitted in the dorsal columns. The anterior corticospinal tract is a motor pathway.

10. c. **Transforming growth factors.**
Bone morphogenetic proteins (BMPs) are multifunctional growth factors that belong to the transforming growth factor beta (TGF-β) superfamily.

11. a. **Parathyroid hormone (PTH) acts directly on osteoclasts to stimulate bone resorption via carbonic anhydrase.**
PTH is an 84-amino-acid peptide, produced by the chief cells of the parathyroid glands. Its overall effect is to increase serum calcium levels, by action in the kidney (stimulation of hydroxylation of 25(OH)-vitamin D3 and increased reabsorption of filtered calcium) and in bone (bone resorption). It acts indirectly on osteoclasts via a secondary messenger mechanism via osteoblasts.

12. c. $Ca_{10} (PO_4)_6 (OH)_2$.
Calcium hydroxyapatite ($Ca_{10} (PO_4)_6 (OH)_2$) forms part of the inorganic component of the bone matrix and gives it compressive strength.

13. c. **Adequate stride length.**
The five prerequisites of gait according to Gage are:

  Stability in stance
  Adequate step length
  Clearance in swing phase
  Foot prepositioning
  Conservation of energy

Step length is the horizontal distance between foot contact to the next contralateral foot contact, as opposed to stride length which is the distance between foot contact to the next ipsilateral foot contact.

14. e. **A bilateral above knee amputee (AKA) requires 80% increase in energy expenditure for ambulation.**
Unilateral BKA necessitates a 25–50% increase in energy expenditure. Bilateral AKA requires >200% increase.

15. c. **It exhibits a high Young's modulus.**
PMMA or bone cement is used widely in orthopaedics, principally with implants. It is strongest in compression, but its disadvantages include its poor tensile and sheer strengths. Its Young's modulus is comparatively low (see question 18), and is between that of cortical and cancellous bone.

16. d. **10.**

	1 point	2 points	3 points
Site	Upper limb	Lower limb	Pertrochanteric
Size	<1/3 diameter	1/3–2/3	>2/3
Symptoms	Mild	Moderate	Functionally limiting
Lesion type	Blastic	Mixed	Lytic

One way to help commit this scoring system to memory is just to remember the worst case scenario; a patient with a large, lytic, pertrochanteric lesion whose pain is preventing them from walking. In Mirels' paper, a score of 9 gave a fracture risk of 33% (compared to 15% with a score of 8) and he therefore concluded that a score of 9 or greater should indicate the need for prophylactic fixation.

17. e. **Eccentric contraction of gastro-soleus occurs during the second rocker.**
During the first rocker the ankle dorsiflexors are undergoing eccentric contraction to control the foot and prevent foot-slap after heel-strike. During the second rocker the body moves forwards with its momentum and the ankle plantarflexors undergo eccentric contraction to control mid stance. They then contract concentrically to provide power through push-off; this is the third rocker.

18. b. **Cobalt chrome, stainless steel, titanium, cortical bone, PMMA cement, UHWMPE.**

Material	Young's modulus (approx. values in GPa)
Ceramic	350
Cobalt chrome	210
Stainless steel	190
Titanium	100
Cortical bone	20
PMMA cement	2
UHWMPE	1
Cancellous bone	1
Tendon	0.5
Cartilage	0.02

19. e. **The disease should be one in which late treatment is as effective as early treatment.**

The following criteria are accepted by the WHO (as described by Wilson and Jungner in 1968):

- The condition sought should be an important health problem for the individual and community.
- There should be an accepted treatment or useful intervention for patients with the disease.
- The natural history of the disease should be adequately understood.
- There should be a latent or early symptomatic stage.
- There should be a suitable and acceptable screening test or examination.
- Facilities for diagnosis and treatment should be available.
- There should be an agreed policy on whom to treat as patients.
- Treatment started at an early stage should be of more benefit than treatment started later.
- The cost should be economically balanced in relation to possible expenditure on medical care as a whole.
- Case-finding should be a continuing process and not a 'once and for all' project.

20. b. **The zone of proliferating activity controls limb growth in a proximal to distal direction.**

The zone of proliferating activity influences limb growth in an anteroposterior direction which, as the limb has not yet rotated, equates to a radial-ulnar direction in the case of the upper limb.

21. e. **Radiolucent lines in Gruen zones 1, 2, 6 and 7.**

Gruen described seven zones around a cemented femoral stem starting with zone 1 at the greater trochanter round to zone 7 at the calcar, zone 4 being at the tip of the prosthesis. He described different modes of failure of cemented stems:

Mode	Mechanism	Cause	Findings
1A	Pistoning	Stem subsiding within cement	Radiolucent lines in zones 1 and 2
1B	Pistoning	Stem and cement subsiding within bone	Radiolucent lines in all 7 zones
2	Medial stem pivot	Lack of supermedial and inferolateral support	Medial migration proximally and lateral migration distally
3	Calcar pivot	Medial-lateral toggling of distal stem	Radiolucent lines in zones 4 and 5
4	Cantilever bending	Loss of proximal support with a well-fixed distal stem	Stem fracture, radiolucent lines on zones 1, 2, 6 and 7

22. c. Ewing's sarcoma.
Chondrosarcomas typically occur in middle age and have a predominance for the pelvis and shoulder. Osteosarcomas have a bimodal age distribution with a peak in childhood and the elderly. They most commonly occur in the distal femur and proximal tibia. Giant cell tumours generally occur after skeletal maturity. It usually appears as an eccentric, lytic, expanding lesion in the distal metaphysic/epiphysis. It is locally aggressive but rarely malignant.

23. e. The ligament of Struthers.
The leash of Henry refers to the recurrent branches of the radial artery in the forearm. The arcade of Frohse is the tendinous proximal border of supinator. The tendinous origin of ECRB is a potential site of compression. The ligament of Struthers is a fibrous band extending from a large bony projection of the humerus, known as the supracondylar process, to the medial epicondyle. It is probably present in less than 1% of humans, and may cause median nerve compression.

24. d. The thoracodorsal nerve.
The lateral pectoral nerve receives contributions from C5/6/7. The axillary nerve: C5/6. The upper subscapular nerve: C5/6. The thoracodorsal nerve: C7/8 and variably C6. The radial nerve: C5/6/7/8 and variably T1.

25. e. Isotonic.
Isometric muscle contraction occurs when muscle contraction generates tension without a change in its length. Plyometric exercises are defined as a muscle stretch followed by a rapid contraction and is a very efficient method of exercising to improve power delivery. Isokinetic exercises are resistance-based exercises designed to provide a specific level of resistance while maintaining a consistent speed of limb movement. They require use of special equipment such as the Cybex machine. Closed chain exercises are where the distal portion of the involved limb is stabilized – this minimizes shear forces across the joint. They are commonly used in anterior cruciate ligament (ACL) reconstruction rehabilitation.

26. d. Z disc.
The I band contains actin only. The A band contains actin and myosin. The M line is the interconnecting site of the thick myosin filaments. The H band contains myosin only. The Z disc anchors the thin actin filaments and represents the boundary between adjacent sarcomeres.

27. e. **Clinical governance.**
Appraisal for consultants is designed to be a professional process of constructive dialogue in which the doctor being appraised has a formal structured meeting to reflect on their work and to consider how their clinical effectiveness might be improved. Revalidation is the process whereby the General Medical Council establishes a doctor's fitness to practise and with it, the right to remain on the medical register. Licensing is the first step towards the introduction of revalidation. To practise medicine in the UK all doctors are required by law to be both registered and hold a license to practice. Clinical effectiveness is defined as the extent to which specific clinical interventions do what they are intended to do. It is described as the right person doing the right thing in the right way at the right time in the right place with the right result. Clinical governance is how health services are held accountable for the safety, quality and effectiveness of clinical care delivered to patients.

28. c. **The graft's three-dimensional scaffold for bone ingrowth.**
An osteogenic graft contains living cells capable of differentiating into osteoblasts etc. A graft which provides a biological stimulus for bone formation is said to be osteoinductive – e.g. if BMPs are included. Allograft and xenograft have immunogenic potential to sensitize patients. Osteoconductive refers to the graft's three-dimensional scaffold for bone ingrowth.

29. d. **A material that has an elastic limit that approximates its fracture point.**
A material that can undergo extensive plastic deformation is said to be ductile. Hardness is a surface property of a material. The amount of deflection for a given load relates to a material's stiffness. The maximum amount of stress a material can withstand prior to failure is its ultimate tensile stress.

30. d. **Changing to a finer pitch.**
The relationship of the inner to the outer diameter affects pull-out strength – a relatively smaller inner (or larger outer) diameter increases pull-out strength. A finer pitch allows for more threads to grip each cortex increasing pull-out strength. A locking screw/plate combination may increase the pull-out strength of the construct as a whole but the addition of the locking thread has no effect on the screw in isolation.

EMQs

1. 1. **e. Cohort study**. 2. **b. Case series**. 3. **j. Meta-analysis**.
A case study is reporting one case. A case series reports on a group of patients. A case–control study is a retrospective study of a group with a condition and a group without, looking back to see if an early exposure/treatment influenced the onset of the condition. A cohort study is a prospective study following two groups over time, one of which has had a treatment/exposure, to compare outcomes. A cross-sectional study examines patients at one point – a snapshot in time. Sequential analysis and equivalence studies are both types of randomized controlled trial (RCT). The RCT is the gold standard.

2. 1. **b. Standard deviation**. 2. **h. Type 2 (beta) error**. 3. **i. Power**.
Variance is the measure of spread about the mean. Standard deviation is the square root of the variance. Standard error of the mean measures how closely the mean in a sample approximates the true mean in the population as a whole. Confidence intervals (usually 95%) are ranges on either side of the mean within which we are 95% certain the true mean lies. The null hypothesis in a study is the default position that any observed difference between the groups occurred purely by chance. The P value is the probability of the null hypothesis being correct, i.e. that any difference occurred by chance. A type 1 (alpha) error is finding a difference where none exists, i.e. falsely rejecting the null hypothesis. A type 2 (beta) error occurs where one fails to find a difference when one actually exists, i.e. incorrectly accepting the null hypothesis. This commonly occurs with low sample sizes, hence the relationship with power. Power = 1 − type 2 error; we often use a power of 80% which means we are happy to accept a 20% chance of a type 2 error.

3. 1. **c. Galvanic**. 2. **e. Fretting**. 3. **d. Crevice**.
Passivation is the process by which some materials (e.g. titanium) form an oxide layer on their surface which acts as a barrier to corrosion. Uniform attack occurs with all metals where their surface is in contact with an electrolyte solution. Pitting is similar to crevice corrosion but the attacks are more localized forming small pits or holes. Intergranular corrosion occurs due to impurities in the granular structure of metals. Corrosion occurs at the boundaries between grains. Inclusion corrosion occurs due to impurities on the surface of metals. Fatigue corrosion is demonstrated by the increased corrosion damage that occurs when metals are repeatedly stressed in a corrosive environment.

4. 1. **b. Proliferative zone**. 2. **a. Reserve zone**. 3. **a. Reserve zone**.
There are a numbers of growth disorders which affect the physis, and in doing so affect a particular layer. These include:
Reserve zone
  Pseudoachondroplasia
  Kneist syndrome
  Gaucher's disease
  Diastrophic dysplasia
Proliferative zone
  Gigantism
  Achondroplasia

Hypertrophic zone (maturation, degenerative, provisional calcification)

Mucopolysaccharidoses

Osteomalacia

Rickets

Enchondroma

Slipped upper femoral epiphysis

Physeal fractures

5. 1. **h. F response**. 2. **f. Somatosensory-evoked potentials (SSEP)**. 3. **a. Latency**.
Latency is the time from stimulus to response. Along with velocity this is a measure
of the quality of the conduction. Velocity is distance between stimulating and recording
electrodes divided by time. Amplitude is the size of the response; a measure of the quantity
of axons. SNAP is the antidromic (distal to proximal) conduction along the same sensory
nerve. CNAP is the antidromic conduction along a mixed sensory/motor nerve. SSEP is
measured in spinal cord monitoring intraoperatively, by stimulating peripheral nerves
and recording the stimulus from the scalp. The H reflex is the electrophysiological
equivalent of a deep tendon reflex. Afferent fibres in muscle stretch receptors are
stimulated, these enter the dorsal horn and synapse with motor neurons resulting in a
motor response. The F response is a measure of the antidromic conduction of an impulse
from a peripheral nerve to the anterior horn cell along with its reflex orthodromic
conduction to the muscle.

6. 1. **f. Squeeze film**. 2. **h. Boosted**. 3. **a. Boundary**.
Lubrication can broadly be divided into boundary (where there is contact between asperities)
and fluid film (where there is not). Hydrodynamic lubrication requires movement (hence
dynamic) which is sufficient to create a thin fluid film between the surfaces preventing wear.
Elastohydrodynamic requires a deformable bearing surface which traps pressurized fluid
increasing the ability of the fluid film to carry load. Microelastohydrodynamic occurs in
articular cartilage where its surface asperities are deformed under load smoothing the
bearing surface. Weeping lubrication differs as a principle from boosted in that lubricant
is squeezed out of the cartilage under compression to increase the fluid film.

7. 1. **g. Toughness**. 2. **i. Creep**. 3. **h. Brittle**.
Biomaterial definitions are important and include:

Viscoelastic – the material exhibits properties that are time and load dependent

Plastic – permanent change in length after removal of the load

Ductile – can undergo a large amount of plastic deformation before failure

Isotropic – material properties do not depend on direction of loading

Anisotropic – material properties differ depending on direction of load

Hardness – a surface property – ability to resist scratching/indentation

Toughness – amount of energy absorbed per unit volume (area under the stress–strain curve)

Brittle – little capacity to undergo plastic deformation prior to failure

Creep – deformation of material under constant load over time

Stress relaxation – with a constant strain, stress decreases

Hysteresis – the stress–strain curve is different during loading and unloading. Energy is
lost (usually as heat) due to internal friction with the material

8. 1. **h. *Vibrio vulnificus*.** 2. **b. *Streptococcus viridans*.** 3. **a. *Pasteurella multocida*.**
Pasteurella multocida is seen with cat and dog bites. *Streptococcus viridans* is seen with human bites (e.g. punching injuries), along with *Eikenella corrodens*. Group A streptococcus may be seen with cellulitis or necrotizing fasciitis, and *Clostridium perfringens* is associated with gas gangrene. *Mycobacterium marinarum* results in an indolent infection and is seen in fishmongers. *Vibrio vulnificus* is waterborne but is a more aggressive pathogen.

9. 1. **h. Hypophosphatasia.** 2. **g. Paget's disease.** 3. **f. Renal osteodystrophy.**
Hypophosphatasia is an autosomal recessive disorder associated with low levels of alkaline phosphatase. Urine analysis reveals increased phosphoethanolamine. Paget's disease of bone is a disorder of abnormal bone turnover. Investigations would reveal raised serum alkaline phosphatase and acid phosphatase, and raised urine hydroxyproline and collagen-derived cross-linked peptides. Renal osteodystrophy covers a group of disorders of bone mineral metabolism seen in chronic renal failure; the 'rugger-jersey' spine is from lucent and dense bands as a result of osteosclerosis.

10. 1. **d. Marfan's.** 2. **e. Multiple hereditory exostoses.** 3. **b. Duchenne's muscular dystrophy.**
A number of defective genes or proteins have now been linked with disorders and included:

    Achondroplasia – Fibroblast growth factor receptor 3
    Duchenne's muscular dystrophy – Dystrophin
    Osteogenesis imperfecta – Type I collagen
    Marfan's – Fibrillin
    Multiple hereditory exostoses – EXT1/EXT2
    Pseudoachondroplasia – Cartilage oligomeric matrix protein (COMP)
    Multiple epiphyseal dysplasia – COMP
    Hypophosphataemic rickets – PEX
    Diastrophic dysplasia – Sulphate transporter

11. 1. **h. Bonferonni correction.** 2. **a. Student's t-test.** 3. **d. Pearson correlation.**
A detailed knowledge of each statistical test is not required, but it is important to appreciate their uses. The tests are chosen based on the data and number of groups:

	Parametric data	Non-parametric data	Nominal data
Two different groups	Unpaired t test	Mann–Whitney U test	Chi-squared test
Two matched groups	Paired t test	Wilcoxon signed rank test	McNemar's test
More than two different groups	ANOVA	Kruksal–Wallis test	Chi-squared test
More than two matched groups	Repeated measures ANOVA	Friedman test	Cochrane Q test
Quantify association between two variables	Pearson correlation	Spearman correlation	Contingency coefficients

Bonferonni correction is performed to reduce the risk of a type 1 error when performing multiple tests. The Kaplan-Meier is a method of survival analysis, used often with joint replacement implants.

12. 1. **d. Plasma spraying**. 2. **f. Annealing**. 3. **b. Sintering**.
Direct compression moulding and ram extrusion are two processes used in the manufacture of polyethylene implants. Direct compression moulding achieves better consolidation of ultra-high-molecular-weight polyethylene (UHMWPE) resin and hence improved mechanical properties. Shot blasting is a method of surface treatment which induces surface roughness. Annealing involves heating a material (polyethylene) to just below its melting point. This is done in the case of UHMWPE in order to reduce the amount of free radicals created during the process of irradiation to produce high crosslinking. Cold working is a process whereby deformation of a material results in increased strength. With regards to orthopaedic materials cold working typically increases both yield strength and ultimate strength but decreases ductility.

13. 1. **e. Weight**. 2. **g. Friction**. 3. **h. Inertia**.
Equilibrium defines a state in which the sum of the forces acting within a system equal zero. A moment is a general term for the tendency of a force to rotate an object about its axis. If the force is acting at 90° to a lever, the moment is calculated by multiplying the force by the distance from its action to the fulcrum. Ground reaction force is the force exerted by the ground in response to a body standing upon it; it is an equal and opposite reaction conforming to Newton's Third Law. The joint reaction force is the vector sum of all forces acting on the joint as a result of body weight/muscle contraction etc. Mass is a dimensionless quality that represents the amount of matter in an object. It is, therefore, independent of gravity. A force is a vector quantity, i.e. it has both a magnitude and a direction. A force is any influence that causes a free body to undergo a change in speed, direction or shape.

14. 1. **e. Superior (upper) trunk**. 2. **b. Posterior cord**. 3. **b. Posterior cord**.
The brachial plexus is divided into roots, trunks, divisions, cords and branches. The suprascapular nerve originates from the superior trunk. The thoracodorsal nerve originates from the posterior cord after the upper subscapular nerve and before the lower subscapular nerve. There is no anterior cord.

15. 1. **c. Ely's**. 2. **e. Ortolani's**. 3. **f. Galleazi's**.
Thomas' test assesses for a fixed flexion deformity in the hip. The Faber test involves hip flexion, abduction and external rotation looking for sacroiliac or hip pathology. Barlow's test attempts to detect the subluxable/dislocatable hip in infants with hip dysplasia. The Fadir test looks for femoroacetabular impingement in hip flexion, adduction and internal rotation.

Selected references

Canale ST, Beaty JH. *Campbell's Operative Orthopaedics*, 11th edn. Philadelphia, Mosby, 2007.

Gage JR, DeLuca PA, Renshaw TS. Gait analysis: principles and applications. *J Bone Joint Surg Am* 1995; 77: 1607–23.

Gruen TA, McNeice GM, Amstutz HA. "Modes of failure" of cemented stem-type femoral components: a radiographic analysis of loosening. *Clin Orthop Rel Res* 1979; **141**: 17–27.

Hoppenfeld S, deBoer P, Buckley R. *Surgical Exposures in Orthopaedics: The Anatomic Approach*, 3rd edn. Philadelphia, Lippincott Williams and Wilkins, 2009.

Miller MD. *Review of Orthopaedics*, 5th edn. Philadelphia, Elsevier, 2008.

Mirels H. Metastatic disease in long bones. *Clin Orthop Rel Res* 1989; **249**: 256–64.

Wilson JMG, Jungner G. Principles and practice of screening for disease. *WHO Chronicle* 1968; **22**(11): 473.

Index